International studies in the history of sport
series editor J. A. Mangan

Rowing in England:
a social history

Also available in the series

Stephen G. Jones *Sports, politics and the working class: organised labour and sport in inter-war Britain*
Nicholas Fishwick *English football and society, 1910–1950*
Richard Holt (ed.) *Sport and the working class in modern Britain*
Patricia Vertinsky *The externally wounded woman: women, doctors and exercise in the late nineteenth century*

Further titles in preparation

Rowing in England:
a social history

The amateur debate

Eric Halladay

Manchester University Press

Manchester and New York

Distributed exclusively in the USA and Canada by St. Martin's Press

Copyright © Eric Halladay 1990

Published by Manchester University Press
Oxford Road, Manchester M13 9PL, UK
and Room 400, 175 Fifth Avenue,
New York, NY 10010, USA

Distributed exclusively in the USA and Canada
by St. Martin's Press, Inc.,
175 Fifth Avenue, New York, NY 10010, USA

British Library cataloguing in publication data
Halladay, Eric
  Rowing in England : a social history : the amateur debate.
  1. Rowing
  I. Title   II. Series
  797 . 123

Library of Congress cataloging in publication data
 Halladay, Eric.
    Rowing in England : a social history : the amateur debate / Eric
    Halladay.
        p.   cm. — (International studies in the history of sports)
      Includes bibliographical references and index.
      ISBN 0-7190-2605-9
      1. Rowing—England—History. 2. Rowing—Social aspects—England.
    I. Title   II. Series.
    GV795.H24   1990
    797.1'22'0942—dc20   90-38505

ISBN 0 7190 26059 *hardback*

Photoset in Linotron Palatino
by Northern Phototypesetting Company Limited, Bolton.
Printed in Great Britain
by Bell & Bain Limited, Glasgow

Contents

List of illustrations   vi
Series Editor's foreword   vii
Preface   viii

Introduction   1
Chapter 1   The professional influence   7
2   The making of an elite   42
3   Defining an amateur   67
4   Little England – a slow demise   108
5   The dominant influence   124
6   The difficult years   141
7   Fusion and unity   167

Appendix I   Boats and style   197
II   Health and training   212
III   The North-East music-halls and the
Tyne professionals   219
Select bibliography   225
Index   232

Illustrations

1 T. S. Egan, cox of Cambridge during the 1840s, influential coach and a major figure in the early debate on the amateur issue.
2 The first of two races on the Tyne on 4 and 5 July 1866 for the professional sculling championship between Harry Kelley and James Hamill of the United States. Kelley, leading, won both. Harry Clasper is in the bow of the nearer eight as umpire for Hamill. In the background is the High Level Bridge.
3 London R.C. oarsmen, 1860. Josias Nottidge is at five in the eight; the sculler is A. A. Casamajor. In the background is one of L.R.C.'s twelve-oared boats.
4 Dr Edmond Warre, Headmaster and then Provost of Eton College, former Oxford blue, a major influence as a coach and determined opponent of foreign competition.
5 R. C. Lehmann, famous coach and secretary of the Amateur Rowing Association, 1893–1901.
6 Dr F. J. Furnivall, scholar, social reformer and one of the founders of the National Amateur Rowing Association.
7 Steve Fairbairn, inconoclastic coach and scourge of the orthodox.
8 G. C. Bourne, Professorial Fellow of Merton College, Oxford, former Oxford blue and sensitive interpreter of the orthodox approach to rowing, with R. C. Bourne, his son, also an Oxford blue and sympathiser with the National Amateur Rowing Association. The third person is E. W. Powell, Cambridge blue and winner of the Diamonds in 1912.
9 Jesus College, Cambridge, winners of the Visitors at Henley, 1932.
10 Oxford University and Colleges Servants R.C., 1934.
11 The Embankment at Putney, about 1880, showing London R.C. Boathouse in the foreground, next to it that of Leander and at the far end Thames R.C. Boathouse.
12 Tyne United R.C. Boathouse at Gateshead just after the Second World War.

The author and publisher wish to thank the following for permission to reproduce illustrative material: 1 and 3 – London RC; 2 – Tyne and Wear Museum Service; 4 and 6 – The Mansell Collection; 5 – The Hulton Picture Library; 7 and 9 – The Master and Fellows, Jesus College, Cambridge; 8 – R. M. A. Bourne, Esq.; 10 – Oxford City Libraries.

The illustrations appear between pages 101 and 108

Series Editor's foreword

The earlier volumes of this series concentrated on the British working class. This volume redresses the balance: Eric Halladay discusses, largely but not exclusively, the upper middle class and its efforts, through the minority sport of rowing, to involve itself, by means of the concept of amateurism, in attempts at both social engineering and social distancing.

In the late nineteenth century, amateurism, as employed by the official organisations of the rowing fraternity, was *inter alia* a means of moral assertion and moral indoctrination. The Amateur Rowing Association, created in 1882, was concerned more with the former, while the National Amateur Rowing Association, created in 1890, was concerned more with the latter.

The internecine struggle between the two British bodies lasted for over sixty years, and few things illustrate more clearly the role of social class in the evolution not only of a specific sport, but recreational patterns, educational structure and moral imperatives.

Undeniably there is truth in the argument that as yet the lower, in contrast to the upper, stratum of the middle class has been relatively neglected by historians interested in the history of sport. However it should not be overlooked that at least part of the history of the lower and middle layers of the middle class is subsumed within, and thereby to a degree indistinguishable from, the upper echelon – partial proof of the latter's powerful hegemonic influence. Halladay provides interesting evidence of this.

Arguably what is suggested most strongly by Halladay's study is the extensive impregnation of British sport with upper middle-class ethical values between the Crimean War and the Second World War. Certainly these values gave rowing its essential identity within the wider culture.

The first four volumes of the series by Jones, Fishwick, Holt and Halladay deal with the social history of Britain. The next two volumes to appear shortly, *The eternally wounded woman* by Patricia Vertinsky and *Driving passions: the hotrod culture* by Bert Moorhouse, are concerned with 'transatlantic' and American history respectively. However, as we shall see in due course, this does not mean that within the series the issue of class relations in sport (and exercise) will cease to be significant issues.

J. A. MANGAN

Preface

This study of rowing in England focuses on one main aspect of the sport's history, the issue of amateurism, its origins, nature and the arguments that it caused. It therefore concludes in 1956, the year in which the National Amateur Rowing Association agreed to dissolve itself and to merge with the Amateur Rowing Association. Developments since then are considered only briefly in the final few pages of the last chapter since more time is needed to see them in their proper perspective.

In writing this book, I owe particular debts to the Council of the University of Durham and to the Governing Body of Grey College for allowing me sabbatical leave and to the Leverhulme Trust who kindly awarded me a travel grant that greatly eased the problems of visiting rowing centres throughout the country.

All club and regatta officials whom I met made me very welcome and some were brave enough to let me borrow minute books to allow a more extended examination of their contents. Peter Coni QC gave me constant access to Henley Royal Regatta headquarters with its more than useful library and records. I am grateful to the staff there for their considerable help as I am to those of the Amateur Rowing Association headquarters at Hammersmith. Neil Wigglesworth kindly gave me a copy of his 1983 thesis on rowing in the North West and Keith Gregson of Sunderland was only too willing to share his knowledge of the north-eastern music-hall performers of the last century, men closely connected with the professional oarsmen of the day. I am also grateful to Robert Rivington who not only made many useful suggestions but who on more than one occasion cheerfully checked references for me in the Bodleian Library. The staff at the inter-library loan desk at the University of Durham were always willing to help and on only one occasion did my often obscure requests defeat them.

The book would not have been written had it not been for the immense pleasure I have had and for the close friendships made in coaching Durham University Boat Club over a quarter of a century.

COLLEGIO REMIGVM UNIVERSITATIS DVNELMENSIS
PRO VOLVPTATE PER QUINQUE LVSTRA
ATQUE CONVIVIIS GRATES AGO

Eric Halladay
Corbridge, Northumberland January 1990

Introduction

During the second half of the nineteenth century a great many sports and games began to become more organise: governing associations were set up and rules and regulations were codified. Rowing, a minority activity compared with some of the others, took the process to excessive lengths since, by 1890, it had managed to erect two controlling bodies. In spite of that unique and odd achievement on the part of the oarsmen, the process made a great deal of sense. An increasing number of people had more time to enjoy games, although the available leisure hours were unevenly spread, and the greater ease of travel reinforced the need for everybody to accept agreed rules for whichever game it might be.

These new associations, however, have been seen as something more than the codifiers of regulations for the field of play. Peter Bailey, for example, in his *Leisure and Class in Victorian England*, has argued that these mainly middle-class bodies tried to exercise a degree of social control by discriminating against those of working-class origin who might wish to participate.[1] This form of social engineering was based on a rooted belief in the virtue of amateurism and of the need to play a game for its own sake. Professionalism was to be avoided because victory became its only reward and the means often used – fouling and cheating – were to be resisted. So too were the accompanying problems arising from wagers, betting and other forms of commercial exploitation. Moreover – and this widened the field from those who played for financial gain to practically the whole working-class – many by the nature of their jobs might find an advantage over those whose work was less physically taxing. Given such arguments, there was a strong feeling that it might be better if those who played a particular game were socially the same as those who made the rules. To be too generous might at best ruin the sport itself and at worst might begin to undermine the foundations of society. Bailey quotes the extreme view of Walter Besant, who in 1887 commented that the middle classes had perceived 'that their amusements – also, which seems the last straw, their vices – can be enjoyed by the base mechanical sort, insomuch that, if this kind of thing goes on, there must in the end follow an effacement of all classes'.[2]

The problem with this line of argument is that it does not always fit the facts and it underestimates the degree of flexibility shown by many of the governing bodies. Cricket preserved the distinction between gentlemen and players until the 1960s but both played together on the same teams. Moreover, the authorities showed a degree of elasticity about the meaning of an amateur that allowed the greatest of them, W. G. Grace, to retain in 1895 the substantial testimonial sums he had gained.[3] But cricket more than any other game kept strong links with its past and managed to retain something of the frankness and candour of an earlier generation. Association Football, after doubts and hesitations, adopted the professional code during the 1880s and 1890s, at a time when the game was becoming the favoured spectator sport of large sections of the working class throughout the land. But there was nothing in the rules to prevent an amateur playing football at the highest level, provided he possessed sufficient talent. In the two games that attracted the largest following by the end of the century, professionalism was accepted as part of the natural order and the presence of amateurs was hardly a matter for comment.

Rugby Union Football, on the other hand, went in exactly the opposite direction, espousing the cause of amateurism with enthusiasm and becoming by 1900 in England a middle-class game. It was unable to accommodate the demands of those in the north for some compensation for time lost at work and as a result the Northern Union was founded in 1895, to become the Rugby League in 1922. But, even here, the position was not totally clear-cut since the founders of the Northern Union only agreed to their players being paid on a part-time basis since they were expected to have some form of a job.[4] Superficially the refusal of the Rugby Union to have any truck with the difficulties often experienced by largely working-class players in the north might suggest a deeper motive, one positively discriminating against those who were not socially acceptable. But it is difficult to square such a conclusion with the fact that there were no obvious objections to matches against Wales and Welsh teams where Rugby Union was in the process of becoming a largely working-class game. The final judgement might well be that the ultimate aim of the Rugby Union was more to prevent the intrusion of the professional element than to exclude those whom some might have seen as socially undesirable.[5]

Athletics, on the other hand, made no such fine distinctions when the Amateur Athletics Club was set up in 1866. Its consitution contained a so-called mechanics clause that effectively prevented anyone in manual labour from joining. This rigid and narrow stance caused unease and heated discussion. In 1879 the Northern Athletics Association, with a wider membership, threatened to boycott the AAC's annual championships and this was sufficient to cause the older body to collapse. In its place the Amateur Athletics Association was formed in 1880 with rules that accepted any genuine amateur, irrespective of class or work.[6] In this case the attempt to impose limitations on participation had seriously misfired and the result was a far wider level of participation than had originally been expected.

The pattern, therefore, was far from clear and the only apparent conclusion might be to distinguish between the theoretical wishes of some of the problems and tensions of the time. Like the Rugby Football Union its main strength was in London and the south-eastern part of Nevertheless, the example of the Amateur Athletics Club does indicate some of the problems and tensions of the time. Like the Rugby Union Football, its main strength was in London and the south-eastern part of the country and in both cases the opposition seems to have been strongest in the provinces. A similar theme was to be found in the rowing world. More significant, the original framers of the AAC's rules were the first to confuse professionalism with the wider issue of social class, seeking to exclude anyone who earned his living by the sweat of his brow. The assumption that those engaged in manual labour might have a competitive edge was taken a step further by the Amateur Rowing Association, set up in 1882. In its definition of an amateur, produced two years later after seeking the advice of Henley Royal Regatta, the clause was included barring anyone 'who is or has been by trade or employment for wages, a mechanic, artisan, or labourer, or engaged in any menial duty'.[7] It seemed to be a rigidly exclusive approach, effectively preventing large sections of society from competing. The only hope for such men was to join an unaffiliated club, of which for several years there were many, or one belonging to the National Amateur Rowing Association, set up in 1890 as an alternative body with a more generous definition of an amateur. The only apparent difference between athletics and rowing seemed to be that, while the Amateur Athletics Club capitulated at the first whiff of grape-shot, the

Amateur Rowing Association survived and prospered. Together, the origins and attitudes of the two associations, but particularly that of the ARA, seem perfect examples of Bailey's thesis. In rowing's case, a superior, narrowly-based group appears effectively to have driven a number of possible participants out of the mainstream, discouraging them from competition except at the most perfunctory level.

Such a conclusion, however, would be misconceived and over-simplified. Certainly at times the committee of the ARA and its ally, the stewards at Henley, could act in a manner that was narrow and even offensive. Their obstinate and intolerant approach following the Great War was such as to suggest they had lost any vestige of generosity. Nevertheless, until the fusion of the two rowing associations in 1956, much of the ARA's energy was consumed in its own internal debate about the place of an amateur sport in society in the light of its own particular inheritance. That legacy was a rich and powerful one whose origins were to be found at Oxford and Cambridge during the earlier part of the nineteenth century. The initial impulse had been the desire of the university oarsmen to distance themselves from the many successful professionals of that time, men whose skills they admired but whose practices they deplored. But their response was liable to be interpreted in different ways. The cult of the amateur could easily spill over into an elite approach to the sport, to be shared with the better metropolitan clubs and public schools. Their specific values and undoubted skill on the water could together produce a closed and proud group, unwilling to admit others to its benefits. But there were others of precisely the same ilk who saw the legacy in wider terms and deplored any attempt to form a closed society. Such men were largely responsible for setting up the National Amateur Rowing Association. Not the least of their perceptions was that they recognised that most oarsmen throughout the country, while lacking in expertise, nevertheless wholeheartedly embraced those notions of fair play and respectable conduct that the elite group assumed was their own particular hall mark. Perhaps the biggest tragedy of over sixty years of divided rule was the failure of some of those in the ARA to recognise that they did not have a monopoly of virtue.

Geography did not help matters. Although there is a great deal of water in England, much of it is unsuitable for rowing. The largest natural stretches, such as those in the Lake District, were in areas of sparse population and, in spite of attempts to hold regattas, such as that on Lake Windermere in July 1810, never proved attractive.[8] The same was true of many other parts of the country. Even the influential student oarsmen at Oxford and Cambridge were forced to devise eccentric ways of coping with otherwise inhospitable rivers. The result was that, combined with the relatively high costs of the sport, rowing tended to be concentrated on three points of a triangle, the two universities and the metropolitan Thames, with Henley as a suitable common meeting place. This concentration of the best resources into a relatively small area served only to reinforce the elite principle.\The opposition, if such a term can be applied to the suppliants that did not belong as of right, tended to be diffused and scattered, the NARA's influence being concentrated into small, separated areas. In spite of the railways, few provincial clubs could afford to exploit their benefits and remained essentially limited in their horizons. So, paradoxically, were the small group of elite clubs within the ARA. Rarely did they travel far beyond limited stretches of the Isis, Cam and the Thames and this only served to confirm their isolated position among many other oarsmen in the country.

There was one exception to this. Against the advice of the ARA committee and with only the reluctant support of the Henley stewards, many of the elite group were anxious to test their strength against foreign competition. The foreign dimension was to prove crucial in preventing the ARA from following too rigid an approach and was probably more important than the domestic scene in forcing a more liberal attitude to be adopted. It was the prospect of international rowing that was the origin of the ARA itself and the need to accommodate foreign oarsmen at Henley largely dictated the amateur definition of 1884. That, in spite of much tension, both Henley and the ARA were able to adapt to such requirements and to make concessions proved in the long run to be to the benefit of all those who remained outside the select sanctum. The sadness was that it took so long.

It remains a complex story, one in which it is easy to seek out villains and to perceive martyrs. Perhaps because it was such a minority sport and, except when the professionals were at the height of their consider-able powers, one rarely able to attract a large popular following, rowing remained isolated, still even in the inter-war years fighting battles that elsewhere had almost been forgotten. But the heart of the matter remained the concept of the amateur: men worried and fought over its exact meaning but that it was worth struggling for was never in doubt.

Notes

1 Peter Bailey, *Leisure and Class in Victorian England: Rational Recreations and the Contest for Control, 1830–1855* (London, 1978), *passim* but especially chapters 4 and 5. The extent and pattern of working-class leisure time runs to no fixed pattern except that, after the 1870s, an increasing number enjoyed more free hours. Legislation in the main applied to the traditional heavy industries and took far longer to affect those such as clerks, shop-workers and farm-labourers. Nevertheless, many employers reacted positively without need of acts of parliament, although such attitudes were unevenly spread. (See F. M. L. Thompson, *The Rise of Respectable Society* (London, 1988), pp. 272–7.)

2 *Ibid.*, p. 105.

3 Tony Mason, *Sport in Britain* (London, 1988), p. 43.

4 *Ibid.*, p. 39.

5 On the debate on these games, see J. Walvin, *The People's Game* (London, 1975), T. Mason, *Association Football and English Society, 1863–1915*, (Sussex, 1980), Eric Dunning and Kenneth Sheard, *Barbarians, Gentlemen and Players – A Sociological Study of the Development of Rugby Football* (Oxford, 1979) and W. F. Mandle, 'The professional cricketer in England in the nineteenth century', *Labour History*, XXIII, 1972.

6 Bailey, *Leisure and Class*, pp. 131–6, 139–140.

7 R. C. Lehmann, *The Complete Oarsman* (London, 1908), p. 252.

8 'Regattas and rowing', report on the regatta at Lake Windermere, 25 July 1810, *John Johnson Collection*, Bodleian Library, Box Sport 13.

1

The professional influence

Competitive rowing certainly existed during the late seventeenth and eighteenth centuries but on how large a scale it is hard to judge. Contemporary newspapers carried accounts of some races during those years, largely on the Thames, but no doubt there were many more that went unrecorded. Samuel Pepys watched a waterman's match from London Bridge to Chelsea in the spring of 1661 and was greatly disappointed at what he saw: 'But upon the start of the wager, boats fell foul one of another, till at last one of them given over, pretending foul play, and so the other rowed away alone, and all our sport lost.'[1]

During Pepys' time there appear to have been some 10,000 watermen on the metropolitan Thames, ferrying people to and from the myriad staging posts along the river, while in addition there were several hundred lightermen working the barges.[2] Most English rivers were the scene of busy and bustling activity, generations of families devoting themselves to their demands like the bargemen at Fisher Row in Oxford and the keelmen on the Tyne.[3] Those who laboured on the rivers in this way were often independent but closely-knit groups within the community, their work frequently dangerous and their rewards normally small. That some of them should indulge in racing each other was not unexpected, human nature being what it is, but, if there was the incentive of a prize or additional earnings, their participation was probably guaranteed. Such matches were dependent on finding people, normally the rich and the wealthy, interested enough to provide the stake, but throughout the eighteenth century and well into the next there was no shortage of men prepared to make a wager on almost anything that had a breath of life in it. By 1800, rowing of this nature had, according to Joseph Strutt, become a popular form of entertainment: 'It is astonishing,' he wrote, 'to see what crowds of people

7

assemble themselves upon the banks of the Thames as spectators, and the river itself is nearly covered with wherries, pleasure boats, and barges, decorated with flags and streamers and sometimes accompanied by bands.[4]

The oldest surviving race was that established in 1715 by Thomas Doggett for six watermen in the first year after they had completed their apprenticeship. It may well be that this contest for a special coat and badge was an attempt to preserve an earlier competition that was in danger of collapsing.[5] As the century progressed, races of this kind seem to have become reasonably common. Typical were those in 1723 for a prize of a boat and oars given by the Lieutenant-Governor of the Tower to mark the birthday 'of the late King William of Immortal Memory' and another in 1749 between seven pairs of watermen for a silver cup presented by the Prince of Wales.[6] Towards the end of the century, regattas, often associated with the massed splendour of boats described by Strutt, began to be organised. At those held on the Thames in June 1775 and in August 1788, the number of competitors allowed to row was limited and they had to be chosen by ballot.[7] It seems probable that by 1800 many of these regattas were well on their way to becoming established on a fairly regular basis. That arranged at Greenwich on 2 August 1831 was advertised as the fifty-fourth which suggests it was being held at least as early as the 1770s.[8]

Amateur oarsmen seem to have been less active in rowing each other. G. V. Cox recalled that about 1790 'boating had not yet become a systematic pursuit in Oxford. Men went indeed to Nuneham for occasional parties . . . but these boats (such as would now be laughed at as tubs) belonged to the boat-people', while an anonymous writer recalling Cambridge twenty years later stated that 'sometimes two rival boats would sally forth together, not so much for a race as for a splashing match'.[9] Racing in boats and punts is recorded at Eton on 12 August 1793 to mark the birthday of the Prince of Wales and there were enough assorted craft involved to suggest some form of activity on the river was already in existence at the school.[10] A few references exist to races on the Thames such as the sculling match between Lord Brooke and a Mr J. Musters in July 1804 and another between two amateurs from Westminster to Chelsea in the October of the next year.[11] Leander, the oldest of the rowing clubs, dates its foundation from 1818 but it may well be that two older clubs, the Star and the Arrow, from whose ashes it may have arisen, had been formed before 1800.[12] But such slight evidence that there is suggests that, until Oxford and Cambridge began to systematise their own activities during the 1820s and 1830s, amateur rowing was largely spasmodic and that the real interest centred on the matches of the professional watermen.

I

By the middle decades of the nineteenth century, professional rowing had become well-established on many of the larger rivers of the country, the oarsmen from the Thames and the Tyne particularly having caught the imagination of a fairly wide public. Never again was the sport to have such a large popular following and its leading performers became admired public heroes, a few of them able to earn considerable sums from their activities. In 1858, A. A. Casamajor, at that time among the most successful of the amateurs, wrote of the Tyne professional and boat-builder, Matthew Taylor, that he was '*sui generis*, combining the practical skill of the waterman with the mental intelligence of the amateur'.[13] Patronising as the tone was, there is no reason to doubt Casamajor's sincerity. He was underlining a crucial element, one that was to sustain professional rowing throughout most of the century, the mutual co-operation and admiration between men from widely different social backgrounds. Even towards the end of the century, at a time when the best of the amateurs were trying to distance themselves from oarsmen of artisan origin, the approval shown towards the professionals was not lessened. Such men were accepted as long as they kept their place and did not try to practise their skills under a flag of convenience.[14]

Rowing was one of a number of sports that attracted the interests of the extremes of society. Horse-racing was the most obvious but so too did pedestrianism, the forerunner of athletics, as well as pugilism. When Tom Sayers of England fought John Heenan of the United States at Farnborough in April 1860, Palmerston was one of several aristocrats and members of Parliament among the spectators together with what one critic of the event called 'two or three thousand of the worst ruffians in London.'[15] Not only did such patronage confer some degree of respectability on activities that might otherwise have met with disapproval – the Sayers-Heenan fight lasted two hours and almost ended in a riot – but the rich and the noble were a source of income both as subscribers to the wagers and as contributors to the large amount of gambling that accompanied many such sporting occasions at that time.

During the 1820s and 1830s the better-off of society often showed their approval of those working on the water by providing what was in essence a form of outdoor relief. Contemporary newspapers remain full of reports of matches for young wherrymen on the Thames, the prizes frequently being handsome ones. During September 1826, those living in the parishes of St Clement Dane and St Mary-le-Strand presented a brand new wherry to the winner of a race between local watermen apprentices.[16] Four years later *The Times* reported that on the 7 September there was 'an excellent scullers match at Vauxhall Bridge between eight young watermen who had completed their apprenticeship belonging to the Middlesex end of the bridge, for a purse of sovereigns subscribed by the neighbourhood as an encouragement for industry and civility'.[17] Similar generosity was to be found in the provinces. At Warrington in May 1820, the first prize was again a new boat, though the other rewards were less generous.[18] The tradition established during the eighteenth century whereby specific institutions or well-known individuals could inaugurate a match was to continue. The Royal Coburg Theatre, under the patronage of Prince Leopold of Saxe-Coburg, presented a prize wherry to be rowed by the young watermen of Blackfriars and Waterloo Bridges, while Edmund Kean, the actor, started a race in 1825 for pair-oared wherries, again the prize being a new boat.[19] Given the nature of the rewards – and a new boat would be worth several months' earnings – it was inevitable that some of these races were robust affairs, fouling being common and argument frequent. 'At nine o'clock,' wrote *The Times*, 'they pulled ashore and, about half an hour after, our reporter left them in glorious confusion.'[20]

Patronage of this kind had little to do with how the watermen spent their leisure time. In the main it was about work and the provision of incentives to those whose rewards were not great. It was a major reason why a number of amateur oarsmen with City interests started the Thames Regatta in 1843, an event that lasted with some interruptions and changes of name until 1876. They were well content with that first venture since 'it earned a good deal of money to be diffused amongst a class of persons to whom very little is a great deal of help, viz. the watermen of the Thames'.[21] In fact they were a dying race, unable to compete with other means of conveyance more attractive to the general public as the river became more polluted as well as busy with increased steam traffic. But the rump of the wherrymen remained, reinforced by the lightermen whose services were still in great demand.[22] But the uncertainty of employment along the Thames during the second half of the century, in particular the virtual disappearance of the wherrymen, was a major cause of the decline of professional rowing by the late

1870s.[23] It was a matter of concern to the amateur patrons and was the main reason why both Leander and the London Rowing Club instituted their own coat and badge competitions.[24]

Normally the patrons of these events were anonymous groups but occasionally the name of an individual, particularly if he was a nobleman, crops up in the records. Often they simply wished to exploit the watermen as part of some lavish entertainment. The Duke of Buccleugh was one, though in truth there is no hint of the oarsmen objecting. Both the Earl of Kilmorey and the Earl of Carlisle, whose estates contained Talkin Tarn as a rowing course, seem to have shown a genuine as well as a generous interest in the professionals of the Tyne.[25] But more frequently it was amateur oarsmen, past and present, who involved themselves in the arrangement of matches and, more important, in the raising of the often substantial prize money. It was the Lyon's Subscription Room, one of the select clubs of amateurs, that organised the first professional sculling championship of England in September 1831. The winner, Charles Campbell, thanked them 'for the handsome manner in which they had handed over to him the whole of the winning money'.[26] The considerable sums involved account for there being only twenty-two races for the championship in the forty-five years to 1876 when Edward Trickett of Australia first took the title abroad. They were matches only for the most distinguished among the professionals and high wagers were not to be thrown away on the second-rate. Even former champions, such as the Thames-born Harry Kelley, could not find men willing to back them if they lost form.[27]

It was probable that for any important race, the search for those willing to underwrite the costs had to be on a fairly wide basis. But such groups of interested men seem to have existed whenever, as happened on the Tyne during the mid-years of the century, there were a number of good professional oarsmen. *Bell's Sporting Life in London* described Newcastle as 'preeminently a sporting town, possessing men of wealth who are devoted to the support of all kinds of athletic amusements, and more especially rowing'.[28] Who exactly these men were is not altogether clear, but there is some evidence that on Tyneside at least, the masonic lodges were involved. The monument in Walker churchyard to Robert Chambers, one of the most successful of the Tyne oarsmen, carries masonic symbols, while a number of his rivals as well as members of his family belonged to the Tyne Lodge.[29] The list of those who contributed in 1860 to the testimonial to Harry Clasper, the first of the great Tyne oarsmen, also provides a clue to those who were involved. In addition to a number of local businessmen, it includes Joseph Cowen, radical MP and newspaper proprietor, as well as William Hutt, the member for Gateshead. Also contributing was the Honourable George Denman, former Cambridge blue and, through the Thames Subscription Club, much involved in encouraging the Thames Regatta for professionals over its later years.[30] The inclusion of Denman's name suggests that, for the top level of competition, interested sponsors had to be found on a national basis.

Much of the support given to the professional oarsmen had been discreet and, on those occasions when sponsors took offence, the press still tended to guard the anonymity of those involved. *The Times* reported sadly of one unsatisfactory race on the Thames in 1861 between Robert Clasper and Edward Eagers that was awarded to the former by the referee, a member of London RC; 'We regret to say that one of the Eagers' backers conducted himself in a most unbecoming and offensive manner to Mr Ireland.'[31] Behaviour of this kind was almost inevitable when large sums of money were at stake. It may well be one reason why, during the late 1870s and 1880s, professional rowing on all rivers began to collapse. The private groups of sponsors seemed less concerned and interested and the only hope seemed to lie in larger, more commercial kinds of assistance. Both *The Sportsman* and the *Newcastle Chronicle* tried to revive an English sculling championship during the years after 1876 following Trickett's taking the title overseas. The recovery was short-lived, in part because of a decline in the standard of the participants.[32] In November 1880, when an American firm, the Hop Bitter Company, organised a world championship for scullers on the Thames, providing £1,000 to cover the first four scullers, not a single English competitor qualified for a prize.[33]

There was one further group whose assistance was vital in the furthering of professional rowing, that of the inn and tavern keepers along the banks of the various rivers. Amateur oarsmen very quickly formed themselves into clubs or were associated with some closed body such as a university college. They owed a great loyalty to such associations and were proud of their exclusiveness. Inns and hostelries played a similar role among the professionals, often being the place where boats were stored and from which training outings were organised. Typical was the Fountains Inn on the Irwell at Manchester. Owned by a former waterman, it became the base for the professional oarsmen on that river during the 1850s and 1860s, including the best known of them in the North-West, Mark Addy.[34] In the North East, inns had from early in the century provided centres for sporting facilities among the mining communities. Once a sport such as rowing had become established in a particular area, the innkeepers became the custodians of intelligence and gossip. This was true of a great many sports and games, including illegal activities such as cock-fighting. It was normally at an inn that the parties to a challenge match would meet to make arrangements, deposit the stakes and agree together upon the rules and the officials.[35] *Bell's Life* remains full of announcements of the kind issued by one of the Clasper family in 1855:

> Richard Clasper of Whickham, having been laid up in port for a considerable time, is anxious to test his speed alongside of the renowned William Patterson of Skinner's Burn. He therefore throws down the gauntlet and will row him for £20 a-side from the High Level Bridge to the Meadows House or Scotswood Bridge. The match can be made tomorrow night between the hours of eight and ten o'clock at Candlish's, Boars Head, Westgate Street, Newcastle-upon-Tyne.[36]

This was a relatively minor affair with a comparatively low stake, as indeed were the great majority of professional races. On occasions the landlord might provide the prize himself. The owners of the Bell and Griffin at Southwark gave a coat and silver badge in 1855 to the winners of an apprentice sculling match, the excuse for organising it being the birthday of Prince Albert and to mark the victory at the battle of the Alma the previous autumn.[37] Others arranged all kinds of different scratch and handicap races such as the James Hall pairs on Christmas Day 1867 and the Jolly Dogs four the next spring, both being rowed on the Tyne.[38] Minor events of this kind were useful trial races for possible future champions and were the foundation of professional rowing, the lynch-pin of which were the inn and tavern-keepers. Many of them were former oarsmen of note: the landlord of the Boar's Head at Newcastle was James Candlish, former champion sculler of the Tyne, Harry Kelley finally settled in the North East, becoming an inkeeper,[39] and Harry Clasper, while still active on the water, became the proprietor of a riverside tavern and was to continue as one until his death.

The result of all this was a degree of intelligence and information about oarsmen that often served the publicans well. Their inns and taverns were filled daily with men seeking some form of relaxation, drink or otherwise. Some of these formed the inevitably large group of people, women as well as men, who were the hangers-on, willing to place a bet on whichever man was their favourite at the time. The publicans were only too anxious to exploit their gullibility and enthusiasm as long as it increased their profits. In August 1830 the landlord of the Ship Tavern at Lambeth organised a 'Novel Rowing Match' in the hope of attracting extra custom. The prizes were various cuts of meat and the scullers were called after vegetables, a manner of doing things that 'attracted many more thousands on the river than if the premiums amounted to one hundred pounds'.[40] Another at Lambeth arranged a women's sculling match in September 1833: 'The females were the wives and daughters of fishermen,' recorded The Times: 'The *canaille* mustered in shoals, and never did we see a rowing match so well attended.'[41] No doubt the landlord was well pleased with his enterprise. By the 1860s, innkeepers in the vicinity of Putney had become increasingly aware of the very real profits to be made from exploiting rowing events. They began actively to renovate their properties 'to appeal to the public following rowing matches' and they were busily concerned with the erection of a pier near the Star and Garter that could be used by passengers boarding boats to follow the various races.[42]

II

The number of men involved in professional racing must remain uncertain. Only the best could command the kind of boats needed for doing well, although some of the boat builders such as William Noulton and G. Maynard of Lambeth, were already by the early 1830s building up their stock of racing wherries, somewhat finer boats than those used for carrying passengers.[43] It must be assumed that this investment was in response to a growing number of possible competitors among the Thames wherrymen and lightermen. Further north, on the Tyne it might have been expected that the most distinctive of the watermen on that river, the keelmen, might have been similarly involved. The *Rowing Almanack* for 1866 mentions that half a century earlier there had been a race on the Tyne in six-oared boats, each weighing fifty stone, manned by keelmen.[44] The problem is that the term seems to have been used so loosely to describe anyone who got his living from working on that river, whereas the keelmen proper were something of a closed community.[45] It was a dilemma never properly resolved by the various census returns where keelman and waterman became seemingly interchangeable terms.[46] The confusion may well have arisen from the manner in which all kinds of boats were worked on a large river such as the Tyne. Keels, barges and smaller craft carried goods, not just coal, across as well as up and down the river for a multitude of purposes. Harry Clasper got his first real experience of rowing in this way. Abandoning work in a coal-mine, he was employed by a coke iron firm on the banks of the river for whom he acted as a wherryman.[47] None of the first-class Tyne professionals appears in fact to have been a keelman. Robert Chambers, the successor in terms of skill and achievement to Clasper, had been a puddler in an iron foundry, James Renforth, the most tragic of them, had his first water-borne job involved in the demolition of the old Tyne Bridge, while W. Elliott, one of the last of the champions of that river, was a miner from the Durham coalfield.[48]

In the course of time, several prominent professional rowing families emerged, establishing a tradition combining rowing with boat-building, coaching or acting as boatmen to amateur clubs. An early example was the Biffen family at Hammersmith and another which went well into the present century were the Phelps of Fulham and Putney. A similar pattern was to be found on the Tyne. Harry Clasper's son, Jack, became a well-known boat-builder, first in the north and then on the Thames, while the best known of the Taylor family, several of them being prominent oarsmen, was Matthew Taylor, itinerant boat-builder at Chester, Oxford and Eton. The Winship family on the Tyne was in the same tradition becoming one of the best-known boat-builders prior to the Great War. Mark Addy was fortunate in that his father hired out boats on the Irwell for a living so that from boyhood he was able to learn the fundamentals of good rowing.[49] Occasionally a sad note appears as some traded on a famous name. James Renforth's brother Stephen, undistinguished as an oarsman, found himself in the spring of 1880 trying to do two coaching jobs at once, at Worcester and at Stratford. The Stratford club's committee was irritated and demanded an explanation.[50]

The number of professional oarsmen who actually raced was never very large. The lack of suitable water in most parts of the country meant that it could never be other than a minority sport. Nor ought the apparently large number of spectators be allowed to suggest that there was a solid core of supporters devoted solely to rowing. In some places such as Tyneside there was a considerable and genuine following but basically the sport satisfied the needs of many for some form of excitement and entertainment just as horse-racing and pugilism did.[51] What was distinctive about professional rowing was that, encouraged by the acute commercialism of tavern-keepers and suchlike, it was to continue to draw large crowds for upwards of five decades during the middle part of the century. Such an enthusiastic response to the sport was never to be repeated. Nor did it appeal to everyone, especially if the consequence of attending a race was some degree of domestic upheaval. Joe Wilson, the Tyneside entertainer, recognised the point when, in one of his stories, he told of the vexed wife, dragged to watch a match on the Tyne. She complained that she had at least expected a contest between 'decent sized boats' rather than 'one man on each plank'. Her irritation was further increased by her feckless and drunk husband who had 'thrawn his muney away on such daftness'.[52]

Working-class recreations were in fact largely male-orientated, often rough and characterised by much drinking and gambling; hence the importance of the ale-house and the tavern.[53] Some saw drink as an aid to physical fitness but this had more to do with the nature of a man's work than with his involvement in some form of athletic pursuit.[54] What free time these people had was devoted to activities that rarely made much demand on a man's stamina or strength. Once sports involving cruelty to animals had been made illegal in 1835, the north-eastern miners, for example, turned to quoits and bowls, demanding some skill, little fitness but both readily adaptable to the needs of the gambling man.[55] Nevertheless, by the 1830s and 1840s, some change of habits became discernible. While traditional games continued and illegal ones were pushed underground, some began to take a more serious interest in genuine athletic pursuits, often capitalising on the fitness and strength obtained in their work. In no sense was this an aping of similar developments gathering momentum at the unversities. There is no evidence at this time that the working class was influenced by the kind of ideas embraced by the muscular Christian school. If anything, this change in attitude, probably more evident among the respectable artisans, pre-dates what was happening at Oxford and Cambridge. If there was an ideological base here, it was more likely to be found in the ideas of Robert Owen and his associates with their emphasis on the need for 'rational recreation'.[56] The explanation may, however, be simpler and more mundane in that some working men recognised that they could exploit fitness and strength to provide additional income and, in a few cases, escape from dull and repetitive work. Pedestrianism, the forerunner of athletics, certainly became popular throughout the country, so much so that in Morpeth in 1844, the local magistrates tried to dissuade runners by threatening to fine them.[57] By the 1860s a number of commercial running grounds had been opened at Newcastle and Gateshead, coinciding with the period of greatest activity on the river by the professional oarsmen. But these purpose-built arenas were used for all kinds of sports and games. In addition to running, there were quoits, pigeon-shooting, rabbit-coursing and dog-racing, all commercially exploitable activities. The proprietors seem simply to have been extending on a large scale the traditional role of the tavern-keeper.[58] This mixture of different sports and games suggests that the emergence of a specific group among the working class was far from being clear-cut. Obviously the physical demands made on those involved in pedestrianism or rowing were different from those indulging in quoits. But as far as the spectators were concerned, it made very little difference from a betting point of view what kind of skills were involved.

There was, however, one crucial exception to this and it was unique to Tyneside. The professional oarsmen there developed over the years a special relationship with the crowds that came to watch them. The many thousands who were reported as supporting the races behaved much like sporting crowds anywhere, indulging themselves heavily in gambling and drinking in the fashion of the day, encouraged by the owners of the many taverns and ale-houses along the banks of the river. But over and above all this, there emerged a rapport between the oarsmen and their public that was distinctive and special. It was to make the Tyne the most important river in the history of rowing.

The oarsmen there developed a cutting edge that existed nowhere else. It was sharpened by their keen determination to prove themselves against all comers, victory being all the more satisfying if it was against the watermen of the Thames. In these endeavours, they touched a sympathetic note among many living in the North East but especially among the Tyneside Geordies. Largely this was the reaction of an intensely proud area, parochial and suspicious of outsiders. Such sentiments were rooted deep in the area's history but reinforced by its contribution towards the increasing industrialisation of the country whose wealth it did not always share. Paradoxically, such deeply held provincial views were reinforced by one of the region's most important innovations, the steam railway. Far from breaking down ancient barriers, they were strengthened. As far as rowing was concerned, railways not only allowed boats to be transported more easily, so extending the area of competition, but they encouraged the idea of a mass following. The directors of the Newcastle and Darlington Railway were quick to see the benefits. In October 1845, for example, on the occasion of Harry Clasper racing at Liverpool, they organised a special excursion train to carry the sizeable group of people who wanted to see the match.[59] The next year, when Clasper rowed against Robert Newell on the Tyne, the railways provided a different kind of service, five trains carrying 'passengers along the line of the Newcastle and Carlisle Railway as the boats advanced'.[60] By extending the opportunities for the Tyne oarsmen to race further afield and by carrying supporters to wherever they raced, the railways were crucial in advertising not only the virtues of north-eastern rowing but also the singular objectives of the Tyneside crowd.

III

The achievements of these Tyne professionals were considerable and in terms of boat design were to be crucial for the future (see Appendix I). This is not to belittle others, particularly those from the Thames, the foil without whom the Tyne oarsmen would never have made so great a mark. It had been the Thames-based men who had been the pace-setters. Between 1831–57 there were nine matches for the professional sculling championship, all the competitors coming from that river. They had considerable strength in depth and were sufficiently skilled for almost any combination of them to have manned an eight and beaten the best amateurs of the day.[61]

The first really outstanding Thames waterman was Robert Coombes, three times winner of the sculling championship between 1846–51. It was the manner in which he stroked a Thames four to victory over Harry Clasper's crew on the Tyne on 16 July 1842 that effectively goaded the Tyne men to begin their assault on the London oarsmen that was to last for the best part of thirty years. Coombes' crew had been able to mark their victory with some generosity, even giving their beaten opponents some of the stake money.[62] Such confident benevolence was not to last long. A disagreeable argument following a sculling race between Clasper and Coombes on the Tyne in December 1844 was marked by coolness and a strict honouring of the terms of the agreement, Clasper claiming and obtaining part of the forfeited stake when his opponent failed to fulfil his part in the bargain.[63] But by then the Tyne men had already made their intentions clear. On the first day of the Thames Regatta in June 1844, Clasper's four had won with some ease. They rowed in a boat, designed and built by himself, that was of shell construction and keelless. A Thames four, stroked by Robert Coombes, was favourite for the championship though on the second day, stated *The Times*, 'the backers were rather nervous on the subject'. They had every right to be. At the half-way stage of the course from Putney to Chiswick Eyot, the Tyne crew was in the lead, only losing because of some steering problem.[64] But the challenge had been made and the next year Clasper's crew recorded the first of a number of victories by Tyne boats.[65] Joe Wilson, the Tyneside music-hall entertainer, crowed with delight at Clasper's achievements, imagining the dejection of the Thames oarsmen and their supporters:

> Farewell the days when London boats were the finest that were made,
> For Harry Clasper from Tyneside soon put ours in the shade;
> He makes his boats so light and neat, brings out such first class men,
> He licks wor builders, rowers too – wor London's glory's gyen.[66]

Clasper's pupil, Robert Chambers, was the first Tyneman to win the sculling championship when he took it in 1859, retaining the title on four other occasions. He seemed to have been a man who combined skill on the water with natural dignity and honesty, unaffected by his considerable achievements. He had the total goodwill of the Tyneside crowd even when defeated. Joe Wilson echoed this after Chambers lost the sculling championship to his Thames rival and friend, Harry Kelley, in May 1867:

> The name o' Chambers, honest Bob,
> Aw's sure 'ill nivor dee,
> The brave, the game undaunted man
> That struggled hard to be
> The hero of a hundred spins,
> The champion frae Tyneside,
> That kept the world se lang at bay,
> Tho lick't, yor still wor pride.[67]

Chambers was probably the finest of all these Tyne oarsmen, representing with distinction all the hopes and frustrations of the Tynesiders against the capital. George Ridley, another of the Newcastle music-hall performers, reflected those sentiments when he mocked the Londoners:

> O, ye Cockneys all,
> Ye mun think't very funny,
> For Bob he gans and licks ye all
> An collars all your money.[68]

Chambers died early but was almost immediately succeeded in popular estimation by James Renforth, who rowed only once for the sculling championship, winning it in November 1868. In 1870 he stroked a Tyne four that won the professional championship of the world on the Kennebeccasis River in Canada and then, while defending the title the next year on the same stretch of water, collapsed and died. Wilson mourned with the rest of Tyneside: 'Ye cruel Atlantic cable, what's myed ye bring such fearful news?'[69]

Chambers died in 1868, Clasper in 1870, Renforth the next year. Their funerals became public occasions, attended by many thousands, that of Clasper being described as the largest that had ever taken place in Newcastle.[70] Each was given a splendid monument, erected by public subscription. Following Clasper's death, the *Newcastle Daily Chronicle* described him as 'but a lowly artisan at best' but concluding splendidly: 'He took his tools, and his strong arm and honest heart, and hewed for himself a pathway to fame and a sepulchre kings might envy.'[71]

The pride felt in these three men was deep and sincere and, as far as Tyneside was concerned, they were genuine and popular heroes. But there was a sadder, indeed tragic, side to their achievements, illustrating the very considerable pressures under which they rowed. Harry Clasper's last race was in May 1867 when he was beaten by a much younger opponent. He was at the time fifty-seven years old and was to die three years later.[72] Chambers' last race was on the Tyne, also in May 1867, against the Thames oarsmen, Harry Kelley, his old opponent. Kelley's easy victory was a hollow one since Chambers was already suffering from the effects of tuberculosis.[73] Renforth emerged quite suddenly, winning the sculling championship in 1868 within a year of his first making his mark. He died three years later. During that short period, he earned from his rowing a minimum of just over £1,500 and took part in forty-five races, thirty-two of them as a sculler, winning thirty-nine of the total. An average of about one race per month, excluding heats, over some three years or so may not seem burdensome enough to lead to premature death; yet that is precisely what happened. Mystery surrounded his collapse at the time, with strong hints that 'he had been subjected to some foul or unfair treatment'. Yet a doctor who had attended him prior to a race in October 1869 wrote that at the time Renforth was suffering from a fit, was cold and had hardly any pulse. He was in fact an epileptic and he was advised to give up rowing altogether.[74]

The determination of each of these men to go on rowing and racing was probably in part a personal decision. Renforth knew of his disability but seems to have been anxious to ensure for himself a reasonable future. His background, like that of the others, was humble enough, though his parents aspired to some degree of respectability. He had been employed as a smith's striker, had then joined the army, serving in the West Indies, but his father, sharing the prejudices of the time against the military life, had\found the wherewithal to buy him out. Renforth had then worked as a boatman during the demolition of the Tyne Bridge. It was not a life that suggested any great future nor one he would have wished to return to, especially as he was a married man with a child. His aims were limited but sensible. He showed himself 'of steady habits, and careful in saving the results of his successful rowing, with a view to some investment in house property.'[75] Rowing was the only profitable skill that Renforth possessed and he was a good enough performer to be the current holder of the sculling championship of England (and seen by some as of the world). There were, therefore, strong personal reasons for his continuing his career on the water for as long as possible in spite of his fragile health. The same was true of Clasper and Chambers, although the first suffered from nothing other than advancing years. But, in addition to private ambition and achievement, there was the responsibility these men owed to those prepared to back them and to the large and enthusiastic crowd of supporters who idolised them. When Clasper lost a sculling match on the Tyne in June 1846 against Robert Newall of London, 'the race terminated without a solitary cheery. The banks of coaly Tyne were dumb'.[76] For the Tyne oarsmen, the adulation and the occasional shocked disbelief of the crowd was a unique experience. In every race, each of them carried the prejudices, the pride and the loyalty of what was in many ways an idiosyncratic community. It was a tremendous responsibility but it was also a burden, reinforcing all those personal reasons that forced each of them to go on competing when too old or too ill to do so.

IV

On the Thames and elsewhere, pressures of the kind that affected the Tyne men were less obvious. Nevertheless, and this applied on all rivers, there was tension of a different kind. It arose inevitably whenever competition for money stakes and other prizes were the main object of the exercise; it could lead to unpleasant incidents both on and off the water and to litigation or threats of it. For many of the oarsmen, especially the scullers, the professional foul was an endemic part of a man's armoury, lending excitement to the occasion. Few would have behaved like Harry Kelley in his first victory in the championship in May

1857. Noticing towards the end of the race that his opponent, James Messenger, was in some difficulties, Kelley stopped his boat and waited for his rival to draw level again.[77] More common were the unsatisfactory goings-on in June 1841 during a match between one of Robert Coombes's brothers and J. Lett. *The Times* commented sourly on the affair: 'If a waterman's wager be the best method of ascertaining which is the better man, and the work of yesterday be taken as one example of it, the sooner such a system is abolished the better. It was a succession of fouling and spurting.'[78]

There seemed little chance of such advice being followed since fouling and boisterous behaviour had been part of the professional scene from the early days. When apprentices rowed each other for a new wherry, the boat was often moored in the river and the winner was not necessarily the first man across the line but the one who managed to reach and physically occupy the actual prize. General chaos often reigned as happened in 1831 at a race off Bankside on the Thames. William Meckett was in the lead but one of his rivals, Richard Harris, jumped off 'his thwarts and, with a leap that surprised many, into the prize wherry he was before his opponent . . . To describe the confusion that followed would be impossible. Both men were at one and the same time on the boat, claiming her as his own, amid the tumultuous vituperations of their respective parties.'[79] At a more senior level, the often considerable prize money inevitably meant that such goings-on would continue, especially in sculling matches. Contributing largely to such robust behaviour was the lack of rules governing most of these races. Those that existed were normally agreed for a particular race at the same time as the stakes were accepted. By the middle 1840s some conventions were emerging for the main sculling matches. Each sculler was allowed his own umpire or pilot, seated precariously in the bow of a following eight, who would shout steering instructions and encouragement. In addition there was a referee, usually in a steamer, whose decision was final, assuming he had sufficient strength of mind. During one race on the Tyne in 1845, Clasper was turned through 180 degrees and then did the same to his rival. At the end, Clasper 'extended his arm and shook hands with his opponent, an act which elicited most enthusiastic applause from the spectators and showed that both men were satisfied'.[80] Since both scullers had made clear how they felt and the crowd was in agreement with them, the referee was left in a helpless state, his opinion on what had happened not being taken into account.

These problems were compounded by the rules of betting and

wagering where, as with the procedure over racing, there was no uni-
form system, agreements being made for each separate race. Whenever
there were disputed cases, as happened in 1863 over an event at New-
castle-upon-Tyne Regatta and in the autumn of the next year following a
race between Chambers and Robert Cooper, the arbiters found themselves without any clear precedents to guide them.[81] When arguments
broke out about both aspects of a race, the consequences could be
litigation or at least the threat of it. When Clasper raced H. Maddison on
the Tyne in November 1846, he was so confident that the referee would
award him the race, following a number of fouls, that he did not even
complete the course, turning round and returning to the raft. He was
right in his assumption but the indignation in the Maddison camp was
considerable. The threats of legal proceedings came in the end to
nothing but only, it seems, because Maddison and his backers could not
afford the probable costs.[82] This was not, however, the case in the
saddest of these affairs, the confused match between Harry Kelley and
Joseph Sadler in November 1867 which came before the courts of both
Queen's Bench and Exchequer the next year.

Kelley seems to have been among the most honest of the professional
oarsmen, described by *The Times* as a man 'who, by a long course of
upright conduct, has gained many friends and the esteem of all who
know him'. The whole business was made all the more unhappy since
Sadler had been coached by Kelley for a number of years. Animosity
between them had emerged earlier in 1867 when Sadler had beaten
Kelley at the Paris International Regatta, only to be disqualified because
of a foul. They raced each other on 28 November for £300 a-side but,
since there was a serious clash between them, William Biffen, the
referee, ordered a re-row the next day. The cause of all the subsequent
problems was the professionals' convention of starting themselves.
Biffen was upstream in his steamer in the region of Beverley Brook,
intending to fall in behind the scullers once they had started themselves
in the area of Putney Bridge. Sadler clearly prevaricated and Kelley, in
exasperation, rowed up to Biffen who told him to start the race
immediately. Nobody saw fit to inform Sadler of the order. Kelley then
rowed over, his opponent following after a lapse of time, only to find
that Kelley had been given the prize. Sadler promptly sued the stakehol-
ders. In the course of the trials, one of the judges regretted that such
matters could not be settled on the water rather than in a court of law;
nevertheless, the case was decided in favour of Sadler on the grounds
that the referee had not made his intentions clear to both scullers

equally. Among those giving evidence, mainly in favour of Sadler, were T. S. Egan, former Cambridge cox and coach and rowing editor of *Bell's Life*, Frank Willan, that year's president at Oxford, and Herbert Playford of London RC.[83]

The interest in the case was considerable but it is not altogether clear that it had any obvious beneficial results. Incidents were to continue and, as happened over a relatively minor match on the Tyne in August 1870, could lead to breaches of the peace. A local journalist wrote that 'for the credit of the sport we would rather draw a veil over the proceedings . . . Partisans of the opposing interests all but came to blows.'[84] One unexpected result of the 1868–9 affair was that Kelley abandoned the Thames for the Tyne and he was a member of that unfortunate four in Canada in 1871; indeed, it was into his arms that Renforth collapsed.

V

That tragic race, together with the loss of the sculling championship to Trickett of Australia five years later, effectively marked the end of the great period of professional rowing in this country. The oarsmen and the scullers of the late 1870s and 1880s seem by most accounts to have been less proficient than their predecessors and by 1889 *The Almanack* could comment that 'this branch of the sport appears almost dead'.[85] Instead, it was overseas competitors such as Edward Hanlan of the United States and William Beach of Australia who caught the eye. After 1882, since the sculling championship had virtually become the world title, it was rowed less frequently in this country and, when it was, it was largely for the convenience of a particular competitor.

W. B. Woodgate, writing in 1885, had no doubts about the reason for this decline. He saw the main one to be the virtual disappearance of the Thames wherrymen and the Tyne keelmen, to which he added the apparent inability of those still involved to master the techniques of the sliding seat, introduced during the 1870s. He also detected a lessening of interest by the best amateur oarsmen and clubs in arranging regattas and events that would encourage the up and coming oarsmen.[86] His point about the sliding seat may be correct but the larger one about the wherrymen and the keelmen must remain doubtful since the wherry was already vulnerable to other forms of transport by the 1850s and the keelboats had never provided large numbers of oarsmen. It is true that improvements to the Tyne during the 1870s virtually ended the need for keels since the colliers were able to navigate most of the Tyne's tidal reach.[87] But the simple conclusion that the decline of the keelmen meant the death of professional rowing on that river, although superficially attractive, appears unlikely.

The answer must be found elsewhere and the argument has to embrace all the main rivers of the country, although the collapse on the Tyne was the most dramatic. Woodgate may be nearer the mark when he explains how amateurs, often with strong City connections, began to loose interest in sponsoring professional regattas during the 1870s and 1880s. One reason may have been the low standard of those competing. He recalled how H. H. Playford of London RC used to run what were called 'Sons of the Thames' regattas in old-fashioned racing wherries to encourage the young watermen scullers and he contrasted such efforts with those of Walter and Harry Chinnery in 1881 when they provided generously large prizes of £1,000 but organised the races in the wrong kind of boats.[88] There was a growing disenchantment between the professionals and those leading amateurs who had willingly over the years given both of their time and their money to encourage this side of the sport. This seems to have been a compound of irritation and despair on the part of the amateurs at a new generation who took to the water, claimed Woodgate, 'for what they can make out of it, by racing on it. Their one ambition is to race and to run before they can decently walk.'[89] For years the amateurs had admired the skills of the professionals even if, at the same time, they had growing reservations about their lax and over-rough methods of racing. But, by the last two decades of the century, the pace of the best amateur scullers and oarsmen was such that they had no need to look elsewhere for advice and instruction and there seemed little profit left in encouraging the professionals.

Just as amateur patronage was being withdrawn from watermen's rowing, the enthusiastic crowds that had once lined the banks were beginning to find alternative sources of interest, the most important being association football. In 1872 the Football Association Cup was inaugurated and in 1883 Blackburn Olympic beat the Old Etonians in the final, the first northern team to win the trophy, the Blackburn eleven consisting almost totally of working-class players.[90] In 1888 the Football League was started, marking a recognition that professionalism was becoming a vital element in the game.[91] By 1888 there were 1,000 clubs of various different degrees of expertise affiliated to the FA and football was well on the way to becoming an attractive proposition to working-class spectators as well as a business of increasing importance commercially. It was significant that many of those elements that had earlier been interested in professional rowing were now closely involved with football. In 1865, for example, eleven out of the thirteen clubs in Sheffield were based on public houses, while it was publicans, hoteliers and small businessmen who formed the majority of the directors of forty-six professional clubs between 1885–1915, the very kind of men who, for example in Newcastle, had once interested themselves in professional rowing.[92] Just as important, although the erection of stands for the large clubs was an expensive business, the cost of a hastily arranged game on a field or a piece of waste ground was negligible for those anxious to play. At a grass-roots level and within the larger community of village, town or city, football was an ideal game, enabling people to identify with a particular team and to form a cohesive and fiercely partisan element of support.

In the face of this development, especially strong in the north of England, professional rowing as a spectator sport had little chance of survival. By its nature it could accommodate fewer participants and, except when fouling was particularly vicious, it was less exciting to watch. Once the interest of the betting public was transferred elsewhere, professional rowing was at risk and, without the stimulus of large crowds, it became a dull affair. The years just before and after the Great War saw a momentary revival, especially on the Thames. The race for the Doggett's Coat and Badge continued annually and there were similar ones at Putney and at Kingston. *The Sportsman* went on supporting an English sculling championship until 1919 and a not very successful attempt was made to revive the series during the 1930s.[93] A number of good scullers emerged from this system. Ernest Barry was the world sculling champion in 1912, 1913, 1914 and 1920 and his nephew, H. A. Barry, took the title in 1927 as did Eric Phelps on three occasions between 1930 and 1933. There were enough competent scullers around on the Thames to produce an entry of 125 for a celebratory handicap to mark H. A. Barry's success in 1927. Four years earlier, fifty-four crews had raced for the Hammersmith Christmas Fours.[94] All this suggests a certain vigour as well as a continued interest by potential sponsors if they thought the cause was worthy enough. When Ernest Barry needed £2,000 to race in Australia in 1920, the money was quickly found through public subscriptions.[95]

Nevertheless the professional scene during the inter-war years differed significantly from what it had been fifty or so years earlier. The most obvious change was the virtual absence of the kind of deliberate fouling that had so characterised the matches of an earlier generation.

Newspaper reports rarely mention it except in the case of an obvious accident and it seems likely that the professionals had absorbed many of the attitudes of the amateurs of the day. Nor does there seem to have been much of a living in the sport, winning at rowing simply supplementing the normal wages earned as a boatman or a boat-builder. It was a matter of some comment that, apart from seeking the advice of their own professional boatmen, employed in the main to effect repairs, few amateur clubs used these men as coaches. The result was that a number of them found fruitful employment abroad, often looking after crews of international standard.[96] But by the 1920s and 1930s this was a sensitive matter among amateurs and it was unlikely that there would have been much official encouragement to the idea of employing any of them full-time for their coaching ability.

Elsewhere, and particularly on the Tyne, there was no revival, however temporary, comparable to that on the Thames. By the eve of the Great War, a number of professional clubs had been founded in the North East. Typical was the Wansbeck RC, founded in 1911 at the small mining town of Cambois in Northumberland. Most of its members worked at the local pit but numbers were never large. The entrance fee was half-a-crown and the weekly subscription was threepence per head. It gained some respectability, if little apparent financial help, by having the local rector as its president and his curate as one of the vice-presidents.[97] Nearby were two similar clubs, Blyth and Southwick, while there were a number of others on the Tyne – Empire RC, Hawthorn, Walker, Wallsend and Gateshead and District. Further to the south on the Wear, South Hylton and Chester-le-Street both had professional clubs and there was another on the River Tees. In no sense were these oarsmen able to make a living wage out of their rowing. In the summer of 1912, the Wansbeck committee agreed to pay the train fares of the two crews rowing in the professional event at Durham Regatta and to contribute half-a-crown towards the entrance fees if they were over five shillings. But it was made clear that if either of them won – and one did – its members must repay the money given.[98]

For clubs of this kind, existence was a mixture of penury and pride. Much effort was put into fund-raising and the minutes of the Wansbeck club are more full of arrangements for dances, dinners and lotteries than they are of rowing matters. After the Great War, efforts to increase income were combined with the organisation of local handicap races but, in spite of all that was done, the club never did better than balancing its books.[99] But, on occasions, there was legitimate pleasure as when the

Wansbeck crew won the Oxo Cup for the first time in 1919, a trophy for professional fours in the North East.[100] It was one of the three main events of the calendar, the others being the handicap fours at Durham and the other the Newcastle Christmas Handicap for scullers that lasted until 1938. This last was an echo of the great period of Tyne rowing and on occasions attracted entries from far afield. H. A. Barry rowed in it twice, on the second occasion in 1933 being the first man ever to win from scratch.[101]

Barry was to appear once more on the Tyne as the stroke of a Barnes four that raced a Tyne crew in June 1939. It was an attempt to revive the old rivalry between the two rivers and every effort was made to make it something of an occasion. Lord Iveagh, a former winner of the Wingfield Sculls, the amateur championship of England, gave the Barnes crew a new set of oars for the race and the umpire was H. C. Bucknall, a former Oxford blue who had stroked the winning British eight at the 1908 Olympic Regatta.[102] The Barnes four won without much difficulty, both crews rowing in clinker-built boats, almost as if they had forgotten the splendid kind of craft of almost a hundred years earlier, built by Clasper. It was a sad commentary on the manner in which professional rowing had declined and, probably correctly, efforts to continue such matches failed with the outbreak of the Second World War.[103] It was just as well since attempts to revive the glories of yesteryear were unlikely to succeed in very different social conditions.

VI

During those decades of the nineteenth century when the professional oarsmen attracted so much attention, the role of the amateur was less clear. Although the patronage of the wealthy towards the watermen was crucial, it is far from certain before the 1850s that those who dispensed it could match in skill and speed those they tried to help. An aspiring blue in Henry Kingsley's novel, *Ravenshoe*, set during the period of the Crimean War, wished he could row as well as a waterman. His discouraging friend thought that with six or seven years' practice he might do so, 'at least . . . as well as some of the second-rate ones'.[104]

Two groups of amateurs were emerging by the middle of the nineteenth century. One, drawn from the undergraduates at Oxford and Cambridge and reinforced by boys from such schools as Eton and Westminster, was in the process of developing an almost segregated pattern of rowing which, for reasons peculiar to themselves, increasingly tried to distance itself from professional practices and methods. The other, with its main strength on the Thames, was drawn from what *Bell's Life* in 1824 called 'aquatic amateurs of rank', a relaxed and uninhibited group often closely connected with the professionals as patrons and sponsors.[105] By the middle years of the century, however, it had become less easy to categorise men in this way. E. D. Brickwood in 1866 reflected on the dilemma that he believed faced many amateur rowing clubs, one that was to mark the development of rowing in England for the best part of a century. As class definitions appeared to be becoming more closely refined, he argued that, although it was often difficult to draw lines of demarcation between this man and the next, every effort should be made to do so. He regretted that 'several so-called gentlemen amateur clubs contain members who are really and truly tradesmen in the literal sense of the term – though perhaps not working mechanics – but who, by reason of belonging to the clubs in question, are eligible to compete with amateurs who are gentlemen by birth, profession, or education'.[106] The extent and source of a man's income as well as his education, the emphasis on the last being on where he had gone to school rather than on what he had learned, were becoming the yardsticks by which social status was judged. The Report of the Clarendon Commission in 1864 on the major public schools had had the effect of advertising the virtues of these schools as much as their vices to those families with social aspirations.[107] But the business of satisfying the needs of the ambitious middle class had already begun. G. E. L. Cotton had become headmaster of Marlborough in 1852 and Edward Thring of Uppingham the next year, each beginning the transformation of a small local grammar school into a public school that, according to the conclusions of the Taunton Commission Report of 1868, might answer the demands of those parents anxious 'to keep their sons on a high social level'.[108] That Report, with its recommendation that parents might be graded according to their educational expectations and means, further forced the pace of change as many previously insignificant schools turned themselves into public schools. They were to provide the bulk of those who went to Oxford and Cambridge for the next hundred years.

That these perceptions of a man's standing in the social hierarchy were becoming important was seen in the degree of embarassment caused to the committee of Nottingham RC soon after it was set up in 1862. Initially its membership consisted of all sorts and conditions of men, irrespective of class or type of work. Hints were clearly dropped and advice was taken; within six months the committee decided to rewrite the constitution. But, warning against the assumption that class distinctions of this nature were always readily accepted, the Nottingham club revised its membership list with some reluctance. It clearly gave the secretary no pleasure and, minuting the committee's decision, he wrote 'that it is with great regret that it is compelled to request those gentlemen who are strictly watermen to withdraw their names'.[109] Some, such as the Northern RC on the Tyne, founded during the early 1850s, seem either to have been unaware of such social distinctions or, if they were, to be prepared to ignore them. It appears to have been a gathering place for professionals – landsmen and watermen as they were called – as well as for some amateurs.[110] The latter may possibly have been what Brickwood called tradesmen, unable to force an entrance at a club such as Tyne Amateur Rowing Club. But it would seem probable that Brickwood was correct and that many clubs, particularly those in the provinces, were not too discriminating about a member's social background. If, as happened with the Northern RC, someone of Harry Clasper's calibre was associated with the club, then interest was likely to be considerable. It was only during the second half of the century that pressures, of the kind seen at Nottingham, led to the setting up of clubs that were based on social status and, even then, a good many seem to have viewed the principle in a broad and tolerant manner.

On the Thames, however, the considerable number of small clubs exercised tight control over those who wished to join. For the most part, like Leander, they allowed restricted groups of like-minded men to gather into what became exclusive clubs. In Leander's case, membership was at first limited to seventeen who met on Tuesdays and Fridays for outings, often concluding with a dinner.[111] The Lyon's Subscription Room, so-called because it boated from Lyon's Boatyard at Standsgate, was rather larger, fifty having enrolled within a year of its formation.[112] Its role in organising the first professional sculling championship in 1831 reinforces the view that it attracted the wealthy to its ranks and the first winner, Charles Campbell, deferentially expressed his gratitude 'to the gentlemen of Lyon's Subscription Room.'[113]

How competitive these early Thames-based clubs were is far from clear. They indulged in private matches, more often than not racing for money in the same manner as the professionals. In July 1829 a four drawn largely from Leander raced another of the Guards Amateurs for a stake of £1,000, an enormous sum of money at that time.[114] Two years later the London Amateurs beat Eton College for the more modest wager of £100, although the temerity of the schoolboys in agreeing to the match 'created no slight degree of surprise among the London gentlemen.'[115] Nor was the practice of amateurs rowing for money unknown in the provinces. In 1840 the Deva Club issued a challenge to race 'the Crusader or any other Liverpool amateur crew for £100 a-side for a race of three miles'.[116] As late as 1855 a Newcastle sculler challenged anyone from Tyne ARC to a skiff race for £30 a-side, though he had no objection to rowing 'for a cup, vase, or any piece of plate of the above value'.[117] Not until 1861 was it agreed to stop the practice of giving the winner of the Wingfield Sculls, first rowed in 1830, the entry fees as stakes of the other competitors.[118] Inevitably in such circumstances there was a good deal of fouling, Leander, in particular, having the reputation for indulging in such tactics, especially when steered by James Parish, the club's professional. His rivalry with William Noulton was notorious and, whenever the two met as the coxswains of rival crews, both the oarsmen and the spectators were guaranteed excitement out of the ordinary.[119]

During the 1820s and 1830s the number of amateurs involved in racing appears to have been small and their efforts fitful and spasmodic. There were numerous clubs, many of them short-lived, where boating for pleasure was as much the order of the day as competition. When the Funny Club organised a watermen's match in July 1825, the main body of spectators consisted of 'the club boats belonging to different parties of gentlemen'.[120] Lewis Wingfield's decision to found an amateur sculling championship in 1830 might suggest some degree of activity in boats of that kind but equally he may simply have been trying to encourage it.[121] Writing many years later, W. B. Woodgate declared that there was little serious amateur rowing on the Thames from the mid-1830s until about 1855, blaming the increasing number of river steamers for making the river inhospitable. Nor was he any more optimistic about rowing in the provinces, regretting particularly the dearth of competition on the Severn and the Trent.[122]

There is, however, some evidence, albeit somewhat crude in nature, that allows some conclusions to be drawn about these early years of amateur rowing. In 1851 there appeared *The Aquatic Oracle* and seven years later *The Boat Racing Calendar,* both essentially lists of names, the latter, edited anonymously by *Iota,* being the fuller and the more useful.[123] *Iota's* inventory contains 971 names, covering 3,500 of their races, all taken from the pages of *Bell's Life.* There are some curiosities. For example, he gives the number of individuals competing at the first Henley Regatta in 1839 as eleven, whereas there were forty-four oarsmen as well as seven coxswains.[124] Again, ten men appear to be listed as rowing in a boat race in 1837 when there was no such match and they are unlikely to belong to the Cambridge crew against Leander of that year since the compiler erroneously gives that race as being in 1835. His references to events at Chester and at Durham do not begin until 1842 and 1845 respectively, although the regatt▩ ▩ere both date from somewhat earlier. On the other hand, *Iota* can be entirely accurate. He gives all the winners of the Wingfield Sculls as well as the names of those who were beaten. Although he does not catalogue the oarsmen at the two universities except for the Boat Races and those rowing at events outside the Isis and the Cam, the list allows some useful conclusions to be drawn about the state of affairs during those early years (Table I–IV).

Table I *Recorded number of individual amateurs competing, 1835–57*

	Henley	Putney	Kingston	Hammersmith	Barnes	Richmond	Isleworth	Staines	Maidenhead	Durham	Tyne	Talkin Tarn	Chester	Manchester	Liverpool	Lancaster	Nottingham	Worcester	Bath	Norwich	Private – Thames	Private – elsewhere	Miscellaneous – Thames	Miscellaneous – elsewhere	Boat Race	Totals
1835																					11					11
1836																					9				6	15
1837																					13				10	23
1838																					4					4
1839	11																				6				10	27
1840	18														9						7	1		1	9	45
1841	29																	1			19				12	61
1842	26											7								11	25	1			12	82
1843	36	45							4				4								17		5	5		116
1844	25	44	1					1			10		5			2				1	12	1	9	2		108
1845	55	54				1					8		5		7	2	18			18	19	2	11	2	16	218
1846	61	63		3	14	4			7	7			10			1	9			3	19	3		7	11	222
1847	57	36			14	15			7	4			4		6		17	3			20	2		14		199
1848	35	26			9	32	17			4							18	9			12	3		5		170
1849	46	17			12	21	24		22	16	2		4				32	13	1		5		1	11	28	255
1850	11	1	15			36	1		20	10			3				12	14			4	2	1	8		138
1851	56					16	8	12	6	12		5		4	4		12	6	2		25	1		8		177
1852	36				34	17		29	6	14			28	26	1		23		10		28			6	18	276
1853	57				25	6		15		32			20	27	14		32		6		14			2		250
1854	57	21				6				29	6		28	26	16		26				1	4	5		16	241
1855	63	28				17				31	1		20	3	9						43	2	7		2	226
1856	71	38	41					1		29			23		17						20				16	256
1857	66	18	62		32		22			31	2		34		20	20					31	2	16	8	16	380
Totals	516	391	103	16	129	181	76	57	55	222	44	158	112	88	33	13	5	199	45	53	364	22	50	86	182	3,800

Source: Iota, *The Boat Racing Calendar.*

The early preponderance of private matches and their continuation throughout the years until 1857 is striking. Including the Boat Race, they represent 16.2 per cent of the recorded competitions. Such figures seem to confirm the somewhat haphazard nature of the sport during its early days and at the same time mirror the pattern established by the professional watermen. Already the Thames was becoming the major focus of rowing among the amateurs, the proportion of races on that river being 69.14 per cent to 30.86 per cent in the provinces, figures closely paralleled by the number of individuals involved, 65.1 per cent on the Thames and 34.9 per cent elsewhere. Henley and the Thames regatta in its various forms – the latter initially had races for amateurs as well as for professionals – represented a solid block but, even without them, activity of other kinds on the Thames stood at 34.7% per cent. It may well be that, given the comparatively high costs of what has always been

Table II *Number of leading competitors, 1835–57*

Universities		
Oxford and Colleges	176	
Cambridge and Colleges	124	300 (30.8%)
Schools		
Eton	32	67 (6.9%)
Westminster	35	
Thames		
Albion	3	
Argonauts	3	
Ariel	2	
Arrow	2	
Barnes	1	
Civil Engineers	6	
Cloanthus	1	
Dolphin	1	
Hampton	1	
Ilex	1	
Isleworth	6	
Ino	3	
Kew	1	
King's College	1	
Kingston	6	
Leander	21	
London RC	41	
Meteor	9	
Neptune	6	
Petrel	4	

Table II cont. *Number of leading competitors, 1835–57*

Richmond	12	
Royal Artillery	1	
St George's	13	
Staines	1	
Thames Club	17	
Triton	4	
Twickenham	2	
Wandle	2	171 (17.6%)
Thames – Anonymous	94	
North East		
Ariel, Stockton	1	
Durham	71	
Newcastle	12	
St Agnes, Tyne	2	86 (8.85%)
North West		
Chester	50	
Lancaster	2	
Liverpool	8	
Manchester	21	
Mersey RC	1	82 (8,44%)
East Anglia		
Bartholomew's Club/Hospital	2	
Guy's Club/Hospital	2	
Norwich	20	24 (2.47%)
West		
Bath	18	
Worcester	61	79 (8.13%)
Midlands		
Nottingham	2	2 (0.20%)
Coast		
Margate	4	
Ramsgate	1	5 (0.51%)
Provinces – Anonymous		61
	Grand Total	971

Source Iota, *The Boat Racing Calendar.*

an expensive sport, this concentration of effort on one major river was closely related to the affluence of the capital and the Thames valley area where financial resources were more likely to be available.

Table III *Clubs and regattas, excluding Oxford, Cambridge, Eton and Westminster, 1834–57*

Thames

Albion Club	1855–6	Meteor Club	1846–55
Amanda Crew	1851	Nautilus	1845–6
Amateurs of Greenwich	1847	Neptune Club	1834–45
Argonauts Club	1834–57	Oceanus Club	1850
Ariel Club	1844–7	Oxford Aquatic Club	1842
Bartholomew's Club	1845–9	Oxford –	—
Cambridge Subscription Rooms	1840–4	Ariel Boat Club	
		Midge Club	1843
Civil Engineers	1841–57	Orion	1850
Cloanthus Club	1848–50	Petrel Club	1850–5
Coldstream Guards	1835–40	Phantom Crew	1849
Cygnet	1846	Putney Club	1851
Devonshire Club	1850	Reading Boat Club	1844
Dolphin Club	1839–44	Richmond Confidence	
Eclipse Club, Staines	1851	Club	1845
Grenadier Guards	1835–40	Richmond Club	1849
Guy's Club	1844–8	Royal Academy Club	1843–6
Henley –		Royal Artillery	1844
Aquatic Club	1845–8	Royal Aquatic Club	—
Dreadnought	1846–8	St George's Club	1841–53
Wave Club	1839	Sphynx	1846–9
Ilex Club	1848–57	Sylph Club, Twickenham	1849
Impromptu Club	1851	Thames Club	1838–53
Incognito Club	1851	Thetis	1845–7
Ino Club	1850–2	Trident	1846
Isleworth –		Triton Club, Richmond	1843–55
Endeavour Club	1845	Wandle Club	1852–7
Sion Club	—	Waverley	1844–5
King's College, London	1939–45	Westminster Aquatic	
Leander Club	1835–57	Club	—
London Amateur Scullers		Windsor and Eton Club	1845
Club	1839–41	Windsor and Eton Hebe	
London RC	1856–7	Club	1850
Merchant Tailors	1839–43		

Places mentioned but without specific names of clubs – Barnes, Brentford, Caversham, Kew, Kingston.

Regattas held, some apparently intermittently, during the period – Barnes, Clieveden and Maidenhead, Erith, Hammersmith, Hampton, Ham and Chiswick, Henley, Isleworth, Kew, Kingston, . Maidenhead, Mortlake, Mortlake and Barnes, Oxford, Staines, Reading, Reading and Caversham, Reading and Thames, Richmond Amateur, Richmond Junior, Royal Thames National, Thames Amateur, Thames Regatta, Wingfield Sculls, Woolwich Amateur.

Table III cont. *Clubs and regattas, 1834–57*

North East

Ariel, Stockton	1850–6	Derwenthough	—
Durham University	1839–52	Dunston Club	1849

Places mentioned – Durham, Newcastle.
Regattas – Durham, Great North of England (1845, 1846, 1854), Newcastle, Newcastle Amateur, Newcastle and Gateshead, Stockton, Talkin Tarn, Tees, Tyne.

North West

Bury Club	1853	Nautilus Club	1854
Lancaster RC	1845	Talkin Tarn	1851
Mersey RC	1857		

Places mentioned – Chester, Liverpool, Manchester.
Regattas – Chester, Eastham, Leek, Liverpool, Manchester and Salford, Mersey, Preston, Preston Guild.

Midlands
Nottingham—

Dreadnought Club	1844
Nautilus	1844
Sylph Club	1839

Places mentioned – Derby.
Regattas – Nottingham, Nottingham Aquatic Festival (1845, 1846).

West
Worcester –

Ariel Club	1847	St George's	1849–50
Intrepid	1843–9	United Club	1848
Nautilus	1850	Unity	1843

Places mentioned – Bath, Bristol.
Regattas – Bath, Hampstall, Holtfleet, Worcester.

East Anglia

New Boat Club, Norwich	1845
Norwich Club	1842

Regattas – Norwich.

Others
Places mentioned – Herne, Margate, Ramsgate.
Regattas – Margate, Ramsgate.

Note Dates are those mentioned in either *The Aquatic Oracle* or *The Boat Racing Calendar*. It may well be that some of these clubs existed both before and after the dates mentioned.

Sources An Amateur, *The Aquatic Oracle* etc. and Iota, *The Boat Racing Calendar*.

Table IV *Professional clubs and regattas*

Watermen's clubs			
Bristol	1846	Norwich	1848
Clyde		Oxford Watermen	
Eton – Brocas Crew	1849	St Agnes, Tyne	1849
Irwell RC	1848	Shakespere Club,	
Manchester Regatta Club	1847	Manchester	
Mazeppa, Durham		Southampton	1847

Note Dates are the years mentioned in *The Aquatic Oracle*.

Regattas			
Bath	1847–51	*Newcastle Spring*	1851
Durham	1846–51	Nottingham	1850–1
Erith	1843–5	Oxford City	1843–5
Great North		*Putney Tradesmen*	1849
of England	1845, 1846	*Rudyard Lake, Leek*	1851
Lancaster	1845–8	Talkin Tarn	1850–1
Liverpool	1840	Tees	1850
Maidenhead	1839–50	Thames Regatta	1843–9
Manchester		*Thames Boat Race*	1850
and Salford	1844–51	Tyne	1843–51
Newcastle and		*Wakefield*	1850
Gateshead	1844–9	Worcester	1845–51

Note Those in *italics* were reserved for watermen crews only.

Source An Amateur, *The Aquatic Oracle or Record of Rowing from 1835 to 1851.*

On the Tyne, in contrast, the generosity shown by local businessmen and worthies towards the professionals does not seem to have been extended towards the amateur side of the sport. Although W. Fawcus of Tynemouth RC was to win the Diamond Sculls at Henley and the Wingfield Sculls in 1871 and three years later Newcastle RC to win the Wyfolds at Henley, these were to be isolated achievements on the part of Tyne oarsmen. The North East may, in *Iota's* figures, have had the largest proportion of amateur races outside the Thames with 12.1 per cent but most were concentrated at Durham Regatta and, slightly surprisingly given its isolation, at Talkin Tarn. The North-West and the West followed with 7.02 per cent and 6.9 per cent each, Chester and Worcester being the leading centres in the two regions. The relative importance of the latter suggests that Woodgate may have been misinformed about the amount of rowing on the Severn but *Iota* confirms his view about the lack of activity on the Trent.

The combined university and school representatives in the list make up 37.7 per cent of the total and this is certainly an underestimate since a number of those rowing at Durham were from the school and the university there. That well over a third of the oarsmen mentioned came from academic institutions underlines the important part that they were already beginning to play in amateur rowing. Oxford and Cambridge and their colleges contributed 300 oarsmen (30.8 per cent) to *Iota's* list. During the second half of the nineteenth century the influence of the two universities was to become even more pronounced and it was to shape attitudes and values decisively for a long time in the future.

Notes

1 R. Latham and W. Matthews, S, *The Diary of Samuel Pepys* (London, 1970), II, p. 101.
2 T. A. Cook and Guy Nickalls, *Thomas Doggett Deceased – A Famous Comedian* (London, 1908), p. 63.
3 See *passim* Mary Prior, *Fisher Row – Fishermen, Bargemen and Canal Boatmen in Oxford, 1500–1900* (Oxford, 1982) and J. W. Fewster, 'The keelmen of Tyneside in the eighteenth century', *Durham University Journal*, New Series, XIX, 1957–8 and 'The last struggles of the Tyneside keelmen', *Durham University Journal*, New Series, XXIV, 1962–3.
4 Joseph Strutt, *The Sports and Pastimes of the People of England*, (London, 1801), p. 70.
5 Cook and Nickalls, *Thomas Doggett Deceased*, pp. 76–7.
6 *Ibid.*, p. 144 and *Gentlemen's Magazine*, XIX, 1749, p. 235.
7 Cook and Nickalls, *Thomas Doggett Deceased*, p. 145.
8 *Bell's Sporting Life in London*, 17 July 1831.
9 R. Brimley Johnson, *The Undergraduate – From Dr. Christopher Wordsworth's 'A Social Life at the English Universities in the Eighteenth Century'*, revised, abridged and rearranged with an introduction, (London, 1928), pp. 195–6.
10 L. S. R. Byrne and E. L. Churchill, *The Eton Book of the River* (Eton, 1935), pp. 114–6.
11 *The Times*, 20 July and 3 October 1805.
12 R. D. Burnell and H. R. N. Rickett, *A Short History of Leander, 1818–1968* (Henley-on-Thames, 1968), pp. 5–6.
13 G. C. Drinkwater and T. R. B. Saunders, *The University Boat Race – Official Centenary History, 1829–1929* (London, 1929), pp. 177–8.
14 W. B. Woodgate, *Boating* (London, 1888), p. 222.
15 W. L. Burn, *The Age of Equipoise* (London, 1964), p. 284.
16 *The Times*, 5 September 1826.
17 *The Times*, 7 September 1830.
18 Neil Wigglesworth, *Rowing in the North West*, (unpublished M.Ed. thesis—Manchester University, 1983), p. 22.
19 Cook and Nickalls, *Thomas Doggett Deceased*, p. 147; *The Times*, 23 July 1829; *Bell's Life*, 8 May 1831.

20 *The Times*, 6 July 1829.
21 *The Times*, 6 July 1843.
22 Harry Harris, *Under Oars – Reminiscences of a Thames Lighterman, 1894–1909* (London, 1978), *passim*.
23 Byrne and Churchill, *The Eton Book*, p. 181.
24 *Bell's Life*, 20 May 1855; London RC, Letter Book, 20 September 1859.
25 *Bell's Life*, 8 July, 1838; *The Times*, 16 August 1858, 22 July 1860.
26 *Bell's Life*. 10 September 1831.
27 Harry Kelley's obituary, *The Field*, 12 December 1914.
28 *Bell's Life*, 29 September 1859.
29 G. Hill, *History of the Tyne Lodge, 1863–1913* (Newcastle, 1913), pp. 14–6.
30 *Newcastle Daily Chronicle*, 6 June 1862.
31 *The Times*, 16 July 1861.
32 *The Sportsman* British Sports and Sportsmen – Yachting and Rowing (London, 1916), p. 426.
33 Woodgate, *Boating*, p. 302.
34 Wigglesworth, *Rowing in the North West* (M.Ed. thesis), p. 26.
35 Alan Metcalfe, 'Organised sport in the mining communities of south Northumberland, 1800–1889', *Victorian Studies*, V. 25, no. 4, Summer 1982, pp. 484–5; B. Harrison, *Drink and the Victorians*, (London, 1971), pp. 48–50.
36 *Bell's Life*, 18 March 1855.
37 *Ibid*, 27 May, 23 September 1855.
38 *Newcastle Daily Chronicle*, 24 August 1871.
39 *The Field*, 12 December 1914.
40 *The Times*, 17 August 1830.
41 *The Times*, 4 September 1833.
42 *Bell's Life*, 29 April 1838.
43 *Ibid.*, 17th April 1831; Woodgate, *Boating*, pp. 142–3, 218.
44 *The British Rowing Almanack*, 1866, p. 171.
45 See Fewster, *Durham University Journal*, 1957–8.
46 The 1841 census described two members of the Clasper family as keelmen but ten years later they were named as watermen.
47 D. J. Rowe, 'The decline of the Tyneside keelmen in the nineteenth century', *Northern History*, IV, 1969, pp. 111–31.
48 *Bell's Life*, 29 September 1859; Woodgate, *Boating*, p. 266.
49 Wigglesworth, *Rowing in the North West* (M.Ed. thesis), p. 26.
50 Minutes, *Stratford-upon-Avon BC*, 27, 28 May 1880.
51 J. M. Golby and A. W. Purdue, *The Civilization of the Crowd – Popular Culture in England, 1790–1900* (London, 1984), Chapter 3, *passim*.
52 K. Gregson, 'When the boat comes in – the songs of nineteenth century sport', *English Dance and Song*, Winter 1978, p. 93; 'Songs of Tyneside boat racing', *North East Labour History*, 1982, p. 5.
53 Metcalfe, 'Organised Sport', pp. 485–6.
54 Harrison, *Drink and the Victorians*, p. 39.
55 Metcalfe, 'Organised Sport', pp. 477–8.
56 Harrison, *Drink and the Victorians*, p. 49 and his contribution to a discussion on work and leisure in an industrial society, *Past and Present*, 38, 1967, p. 101. See also Richard Holt, *Sport and the British – A Modern History* (Oxford, 1989),

pp. 42–3 on the issue of rational recreation.

57 Metcalfe, 'Organised Sport', p. 477.

58 *Ibid*, p. 478.

59 *Newcastle Journal*, 23 July 1845.

60 *The Times*, 24 June 1846.

61 Woodgate, *Boating*, p. 218.

62 *Newcastle Journal*, 23 July 1842.

63 *Ibid*, 21–28 December 1844.

64 *The Times*, 24 June 1844.

65 Clasper stroked the winning championship fours of 1845, 1848, 1849, 1856, 1857, 1859 and 1862. On two of those occasions, 1849 and 1856, the crew was a combined one of Tyne and Thames men, Coombes being in the 1849 boat though 'it is said that circumstances, not inclination exactly, conduced to this union.' (*Newcastle Journal*, 14 July 1849). Other Tyne fours won the event in 1854, 1861, 1870 and 1875. (Woodgate, *Boating*, pp. 298–301).

66 Joe Wilson, *Tyneside Songs and Drolleries* (Newcastle, 1890), pp. 340–1.

67 Gregson, *English Dance and Song*, p. 92.

68 *Ibid*, p. 93.

69 *Ibid*.

70 *Newcastle Journal*, 18 July 1870.

71 *Newcastle Daily Chronicle*, 19 July 1870.

72 *Durham County Advertiser*, 15 July 1870.

73 Woodgate, *Boating*, p. 221.

74 *Newcastle Daily Chronicle*, 24 August 1871.

75 *Ibid*.

76 *Newcastle Journal*, 27 June 1846.

77 *The Times*, 13 May 1857.

78 *Ibid*, 9 June 1841.

79 *Bell's Life*, 3 July 1831.

80 *Newcastle Journal*, 29 November 1845.

81 Argonaut (E. D. Brickwood), *The Arts of Rowing and Training* (London, 1866), p. ix.

82 *Newcastle Journal*, 21 November 1846; *Newcastle Courant*, 5 March 1847.

83 *The Times*, 28, 29 November 1867, 28, 29 February, 6, 11 March, 17 April 1868; *Law Journal Report*, 1869, 38, pp. 91–7.

84 *Newcastle Daily Chronicle*, 9 August 1870.

85 *The Almanack*, 1889, p. 3.

86 Woodgate, *Boating*, pp. 231–5.

87 Rowe, *Northern History*, IV, 1969

88 Woodgate, *Boating*, pp. 231, 234.

89 *Ibid*, p. 232.

90 T. Mason, *Association Football and English Society*, 1863–1915 (Sussex, 1980), p. 33.

91 *Ibid*, pp. 16–7, 72–4, 96–100.

92 *Ibid*, pp. 27, 42–6.

93 H. Cleaver, *A History of Rowing* (London, 1957), pp. 202–3.

94 *Ibid*, pp. 28–9.

95 *Ibid*, p. 29.

96 *Ibid*, pp. 17–8, 32.
97 Wansbeck RC, *Minutes*, 29 May 1911.
98 *Ibid*, 28 April, 30 June 1912.
99 *Ibid*. 21 July 1919.
100 *Ibid*.
101 *Newcastle Journal*, 27 December 1933.
102 *Ibid*, 12, 20 June 1939.
103 *Newcastle Evening Chronicle*, 19 March 1940.
104 Henry Kingsley, *Ravenshoe* (London, 1894 edition), pp. 55.
105 *Bell's Life*, 4 April 1824.
106 Argonaut, *The Arts*, p. 151.
107 M. J. Wiener, *English Culture and the Decline of the Industrial Spirit, 1850–1980* (Cambridge, 1982), pp. 16–9.
108 *Report of the Schools Inquiry Commission'* (Taunton Report), *parliamentary Papers, 1868*, I, pp. 17–8.
109 Nottingham BC, *Minutes*, 8 December 1862.
110 *Newcastle Daily Chronicle*, 8 March 1865.
111 Burnell and Rickett, *A Short History of Leander*, p. 15.
112 *Bell's Life*, 8 May 1831.
113 *Ibid*, 9 September 1831.
114 *Ibid*, 4 July 1829.
115 *Ibid*, 24 July 1831.
116 Wigglesworth, *Rowing in the North West*, (M.Ed. thesis), p. 45.
117 *Bell's Life*, 28 October 1855.
118 Woodgate, *Boating*, pp. 193–4; Argonaut, *The Arts*, pp. 151–2.
119 Burnell and Rickett, *A Short History of Leander*, pp. 10–12.
120 *Bell's Life*, 4 September 1825.
121 Woodgate, *Boating*, p. 181.
122 *Ibid*, pp. 181, 184.
123 An Amateur, *The Aquatic Oracle or Record of Rowing from 1835 to 1851* (London, 1851); Iota, *The Boat Racing Calendar or Record of the Performances of the Principal Winning Amateurs in England and Wales from 1835 to 1857* (London, 1858). *The Aquatic Oracle* has a section devoted to professional rowing.
124 H. T. Steward, *Henley Royal Regatta, 1839–1902* (London, 1903), pp. 5–6.

2

The making of an elite

During these early years, the amateurs regarded the professionals with considerable admiration. Nevertheless, they seem to have preferred that, at regattas, like should normally race against like. The early officials, as at Chester and at Durham, accordingly tried to make arrangements that prevented amateurs and professionals from competing against each other.[1] A man's amateur status was not at risk; that in those days was not an issue of any importance. W. B. Woodgate, the Oxford blue of the early 1860s, was quite clear on that point: 'The old theory of an amateur,' he wrote, 'was that he was a gentleman and that the two were simply convertible terms.' Such a man, he went on, 'might make rowing his sport, so long as he did not actually make it his ostensible means of livelihood'.[2] It was a simple approach and one with which few at the time would have quibbled, least of all Woodgate himself who was not averse to testing his skills against a professional if the occasion presented itself.[3]

Some, however, were becoming less certain. At Durham Regatta in 1860, the officials broke their own unwritten rules by allowing Harry Clasper to compete in a sculling event against some amateurs. His four opponents naturally objected, each seeing his chance of victory fading against the opposition of such a formidable oarsman. They accordingly plotted his downfall. Since all five were racing at once on a narrow river, the conspiracy was easily effected. One of the amateurs agreed to sacrifice himself by ramming Clasper's boat; both were forced into the water and came to blows.[4] The rather sad little incident encapsulated what was to be one source of division in rowing, that between those who simply used their muscles occasionally on the water as a form of pleasure and those who exercised themselves permanently, whether as professional oarsmen or through some form of work demanding physical labour.

There were also signs of another form of objection. The first amateurs had seen no particular problem in competing for financial gain. The Wingfield Sculls were until 1861 a sweepstake, the winner taking all.[5] But well before then the question was already beginning to be asked as to whether or not this was a proper way for an amateur to behave. Some, more particularly those on the metropolitan Thames, could not at first see why there should be any wavering on the matter. When, in 1839, a member of the Dolphin Club demurred about rowing a Leander man for a wager, the latter protested that 'public interest in the river as well as the spirit of rowing would soon cease if all contests were for honour only'.[6]

This particular dispute became the subject of some public debate. Significantly the Leander man shifted his target to the two universities and it was largely Oxford and Cambridge oarsmen who conducted the defence. One wrote that 'at neither of the universities is it considered essential to the "character of a match" or to "the spirit of rowing" that a gentlemanly amusement should be converted to a source of profit', while another, given to irony, stated that if university oarsmen were to behave in such a manner, 'they would never again appear on the Isis or Cam, but must retire to some other place to practise their new handicraft and count their honourable gains'. The perplexed Leander man expressed his disbelief at such earnest sentiments, concluding that 'your correspondents of last week would lead us to infer that he who rows for money is no gentleman, while some may consider that he who makes a public match without some stake is no small fool'.[7]

I

The incident over the Dolphin Club sculler was an early indication of a more scrupulous approach that was by the end of the century to divide rowing in this country into two camps. It was to produce in time a praetorian guard that was not only highly skilful on the water but was able to exercise considerable influence and power. Its instincts were to resist any attempt at sharing its benefits with others. The origins and values of that elite group are of central importance in the understanding of rowing's development in England. Its members could on occasions lend themselves to caricature and misrepresentation. But they were never an entirely unanimous body of men and there was sufficient resistance among them to the implementation of over-harsh remedies to ensure that in the end generosity overcame bigotry. But the arguments were often fierce and nearly always lengthy. Compromises, when they came, too often seemed grudgingly given. At the centre of their creed was a sincere, if narrowly-based, belief in the virtues of amateurism. One of the great tragedies of English rowing was their failure to realise that it was equally important to those who were seen as its opponents.

It is in this context that the contribution of the university oarsmen to the argument between the Leander and the Dolphin Club scullers becomes significant. It indicates that, by the late 1830s, rowing men at Oxford and Cambridge were becoming wary of the attitudes of some of the amateurs of the day. In time they were to convert most of the latter to their point of view, especially those on the metropolitan Thames. This alliance was to be of great import, especially when it was reinforced during the second half of the century by the public schools, increasingly consumed by their passion for athleticism.

Competitive rowing at Oxford and Cambridge only really began following the Napoleonic Wars. Charles Merivale, a member of Cambridge's first Boat Race crew, recalled that, when he first became an undergraduate, 'boating and boat-racing were but as a thing of yesterday with us' but that 'in the third year, 1828, most of the colleges manned their eights, and we warmed to our work . . . In 1829 we aspired to compete with Oxford.'[8] Very quickly a unique rowing calendar was developed, totally controlled by the resident students and in time providing competition all the year round.[9] In constructing this, the universities and colleges were forced to consider their attitudes towards contemporary practices elsewhere. Initially there was an understandable degree of ambivalence as young men tried to establish their own particular conventions. In 1823 objections to some Oxford colleges using watermen in their eights halted the nascent bumping racing and led to a ban on the practice.[10] The business of rowing for wagers also exercised some student minds. On the eve of the first boat race, Merivale felt compelled to write to his mother 'to caution you not to believe an advertisement which is to be seen in some of the papers about the match being for £500. It is not an exaggeration even, but a lie.'[11] Nevertheless, whenever university or college oarsmen ventured outside their home waters, usually to race Leander, they were often forced to compromise Merivale's high-flown principles. In 1828 Leander beat Christ Church on the Thames in a race for £200 and three years later defeated Oxford for a similar sum on the Henley reach.[12] In the latter contest, as well as in the two matches between Leander and Cambridge in 1837 and 1838, professional coxes were used by the rival boats, although there is no mention of there being wagers on the two Cambridge ventures. It was Leander who had insisted on watermen acting as steersmen but, given the known rivalry between those involved, J. Parish for Leander and W. Noulton for Cambridge, the students were right to demand no fouling. The 1837 race passed without mishap but the boring between the two steersmen the next year was of such a nature that the race was declared void.[13]

It seems clear that by the 1840s the university oarsmen were developing some reasonably coherent views on such issues as wagers and fouling. What had originally dragged the Oxford and Cambridge correspondents into the Dolphin Club dispute was the Leander sculler's claim that it was the university authorities who had forbidden racing for money. In their replies, they made the point that the universities, as such, had nothing to do with the issue and that the proscription was solely a self-imposed convention, accepted by all in the interests of inter-collegiate rowing.[14] What was happening at both universities was that the unique system of boat-racing that had been adopted was beginning to impose its own form of discipline. In particular, wagers and fouling were discouraged, a deliberate distancing of the Isis and the Cam from practices elsewhere.[15] The point was made forcibly in 1839. The Boat Race of that year was in such marked contrast to the Leander match of 1838 that C. J. Selwyn, brother of one of the 1829 Cambridge crew and himself a Boat Race umpire, felt that it had established that 'watermen's ways are not our ways, or watermen's notions our notions'. The next year he was even more explicit: 'The principles which we always maintained were: first that gentlemen should steer; second (which follows from the first) that fouling should be abolished; and last, not least, that victory should be its own reward.'[16]

Selwyn's statement was the first attempt to formulate a clear and coherent view about the nature of university rowing. In his use of the word 'gentleman' he seemed to be encouraging increasing aloofness from the leading amateur groups, particularly Leander, whose approach he was condemning as much as he was that of the professionals. Nevertheless, the full implication of his views was not immediately realised. The use of professional steersmen was abandoned and with it the consequent risk of fouling, but Cambridge, especially, were reluctant to abandon the use of watermen in training crews on the Cam. The Lady Margaret BC used one around 1845, while, in the Lent term 1849, First Trinity BC engaged one of the Clasper brothers for £4 per week and his rail fare.[17] Oxford, on the other hand, passed a rule in 1841 forbidding the use of 'any watermen in the capacity of coach or trainer within three weeks of the race', a lead followed tardily by Cambridge only in 1873.[18] But the greatest argument hinged round the use of watermen as coaches of the Boat Race crews. Again, Cambridge was slower to give up the practice and it was the direct cause of T. S. Egan, former cox and coach of various Cambridge boats, becoming involved with the Oxford crew of 1852 which promptly won.

Egan justified his temporary migration by taking Selwyn's views to their logical conclusion. He argued that 'eight-oared rowing necessarily declines from its high perfection in the hands of watermen'. What was threatened, he felt, was:

> that entire uniformity and machine-like regularity of performance, for which the practised eye looks at once in a university crew and which is the glory and delight of an oarsman . . . We ought to be able to point to our match crews and challenge the world to produce anything so uniform in motion, so polished in form, at once so speedy and so graceful, as one of those picked eights of the gentle blood of England.[19]

Egan's forceful plea had been earlier reinforced by his friend and rival, A. T. W. Shadwell, cox of various Oxford crews as well as coach. In his conclusion to what is the first rowing manual in 1846, Shadwell had stressed what he felt was a fundamental issue in university and college rowing, namely the qualities of character that, he argued, were demanded of any sportsman. The basic need was discipline, 'its seven-fold aegis'. He stressed that:

> discipline involves in itself the notion of principles, and these, when carried into practice, enter into men's ways of thinking and feeling, and give a decided bias to their conduct as rowing men. Thus, like any constitutional maxims, they are much more than written law; they are not letter but spirit; and become the hereditary guides of every successive set of men in the boat club, a wholesome pervading system of tradition and a standard which each man endeavours to act up to. Discipline, in truth, has an immense moral effect, and that an enduring one.[20]

II

The degree to which these earnest sentiments were accepted must not be exaggerated. Rowing was only one of many pastimes indulged in by the undergraduates and the rowdy and often ill-disciplined pursuits of the past were not abandoned overnight. Organised athletics, for example, emerged at Oxford about 1850, largely because a few students at Exeter College concluded that running might be a more satisfactory activity than steeplechasing on hired but worked-out horses. Initially they imported all the normal practices of the equine world, including the keeping of a book at the porter's lodge.[21] If W. Tuckwell is to be believed, rowing was 'a mere pleasant incident in a summer term' until the excitement caused in 1843 when seven Oxford men, the eighth being ill, beat the full might of the Cambridge Subscription Rooms in the final of the Grand at Henley.[22] He may well have been right since most sports demanded their heroic moments. As it became more popular on the Isis and the Cam, it would be easy to assume that, under the influence of the likes of Shadwell and Egan, the aim was to produce saints in rowing boats. The rumbustious approach of W. B. Woodgate, dedicated to the river as he was, warns against such a conclusion. As an undergraduate he lived life to the full and seems to have survived in the main because the authorities at Brasenose College, Oxford, were prepared to tolerate activities that they might have deplored in a less talented athlete.[23] One consequence of all this was often a degree of arrogant superiority that had its unacceptable side. Other river users, such as the bargemen, themselves far from mealy-mouthed, found themselves roughly pushed aside. In May 1864, one boatman, having waited at Folly Bridge for the college races to end, found himself set upon by two under-graduates and was taken in charge by the police. Fortunately, in this case, his assailants were fined but incidents of that kind did little to advertise the apparent virtues so keenly preached by Shadwell and Egan.[24]

Obviously as rowing became more popular and larger numbers of boats appeared on the Isis and the Cam, rules and regulations were needed to govern the behaviour of the traffic. Where by-laws needed altering, the authorities normally favoured the university students. The ancient rights of way of barges and other working boats over other river-users were abolished, limits were placed on the use of punts during races and, in a different vein, the senior dons at Oxford warned against the use of outriggers, considered a dangerous innovation.[25] At both universities, the river was ceasing to be a public highway in the long-accepted sense and was instead becoming almost the private domain of the student oarsmen, already, by the 1840s and 1850s, developing their own particular approach to the sport, superior, often arrogant and on occasions loutish.

Nevertheless, writing in 1870, Leslie Stephen could argue that the ideas of Charles Kingsley, Thomas Hughes and F. D. Maurice fell on ground already well prepared for them.[26] How far these men drew conclusions from the behaviour of the undergraduate oarsmen is uncertain but the rowing connections and interests of many of them remains striking. Leslie Stephen himself, while a young Fellow of Trinity Hall, Cambridge, took an obsessive interest in coaching the college boats as well as being one of those responsible for the first inter-university athletics match in 1864.[27] Noel Annan has claimed that it was he, rather than Charles Kingsley, who was the real founder of muscular Christianity, although both rejected the name.[28] Stephen was a close friend of Thomas Hughes and preached the sermon at the funeral of one of the younger Hughes brothers who died from an athletic injury. Another of the brothers, George, twice rowed for Oxford, including being the stroke of the 1843 seven-oar, as well as being in the university cricket eleven. His cox, in 1843, had been Shadwell while the beaten Cambridge boat was steered by Egan. Much of the action of Thomas Hughes's less well-known novel, *Tom Brown at Oxford* (1860), centres on the fortunes of the college boat. Charles Kingsley himself often took his relaxation on the water, startling his undergraduate audience while he was Regius Professor of History by occasionally cutting short his lectures to go sculling on the Cam.[29] The rowing interest of so many of them suggests that an important part of the inspiration for that cult of athleticism, that was to dominate the late Victorian public schools and universities, is to be found among those active on the Isis and the Cam during the 1840s and 1850s.[30]

Such a development was to be reinforced at both universities by changes in attitudes among the dons, not all of whom would have seen themselves as disciples of Kingsley and the muscular Christian school. Reform was in the air, both in the structure of university government and in the contents of the somewhat narrow academic disciplines. One German observer, while pointing out that the universities in his own country were intended to breed learned and practical men, commented that Oxford and Cambridge were content to produce 'the first and most distinctive flower of the national life, a well educated gentleman'.[31] Newman in his *The Idea of a University* (1854) would have endorsed such a conclusion and been happy for it to continue. In a deliberately provocative contrast, he stated his strong preference for the kind of place that 'merely brought a number of young men together for three or four years' over the type of university that placed all its trust in examinations.[32] Throughout the many changes at both universities during the Victorian period, this idea of a liberal education in which a hidden curriculum generously supported the specifically academic was never really challenged. As M. J. Wiener and Oliver MacDonagh have both emphasised, the two universities tried to hold themselves aloof from the competitive world of business and industry, stressing instead that they provided for most students a broad, general experience rather than a specific form of training.[33] In reacting in this way, the dons reflected the wishes of most of their students, the majority of whom still came from a narrow social background of clergymen, professional men and the gentry.[34]

By the later years of the nineteenth century, the universities, abetted by the public schools, had produced a quite distinctive form of education.[35] Some of course deplored it. Mark Pattison of Lincoln College, Oxford, poured scorn on Benjamin Jowett, Master of Balliol, for turning Oxford into some kind of superior public school: 'The separation between Jowett and myself consists in a difference upon the fundamental question of university politics – viz. science and learning v. school keeping.'[36] The climate of opinion, however, was against him. Both universities were still able to nurture considerable and influential scholars but, in the main, most of the students were honest enough men with what Stephen called 'obtuse intellects'.[37] Many would be like Samuel Lodge, in later life a successful grammar school headmaster, who went up to Lincoln College in 1847. After a brief flirtation with Tractarianism, he threw himself enthusiastically into the affairs of the college boat club. 'I wasted my time sadly', he wrote, 'absolutely giving up all my reading . . . If a man liked to be idle, he had a long time before him in which to indulge his tastes.'[38]

It was just this kind of undergraduate whom Leslie Stephen, one of the first of a new kind of don, thought was worth educating. One of his former pupils recalled the debt he owed:

> He had the greatest possible influence for good upon the undergraduates from the very first . . . No undergraduate of my time ever looked upon Stephen only as tutor and lecturer; he was a real friend to us, and sought to form and strengthen, purify and utilise, the characters of many of us. He took the deepest interest in our manly sports. He *made* that boat of 1859 which was the pioneer of all Trinity Hall's rowing successes during these last fifty years . . . He did all this for the ulterior purpose of making men of us and not loafers.[39]

Stephen believed that every young man should have some kind of abiding interest and, if it happened to be rowing, so much the better since he was himself so engrossed in it. He confessed that it was a sport so

> bound up with memories of close and delightful intimacies, that it almost makes me sentimental. To my mind, the pleasantest of all such bonds are

those which we form with fellow students by talking nonsense with them and mistaking it for philosophy: but an average undergraduate wants some more material bond, and I know none that acts with more energy than a common devotion to such absorbing amusements.[40]

Henry Jackson, fellow of Trinity, Cambridge, was another who confirmed Stephen's approach: 'It was the man who read hard, the man who rowed hard, and let me add, the man who did both, whom I and my contemporaries respected and admired.'[41] F. D. Maurice was so impressed by this marked change in the relationship between dons and undergraduates that he told Kingsley how much he regretted that nothing comparable had existed in his own student days.[42]

This was just the kind of environment that allowed university and college rowing to flourish. With Shadwell, Egan and others whom they had coached still prepared to offer help and guidance and with dons, such as Stephen and Jackson to give them an encouraging blessing, it was not surprising that the oarsmen on the Isis and the Cam saw themselves as a privileged group. Insulated by their own termly competitions from the rest of the rowing community, they saw no reason to display their virtues publicly except on Boat Race day and at Henley. There was therefore real pressure to preserve this advantaged position, cocooned and quarantined as it was, the inevitable consequence of the self-confident and patrician views of Selwyn, Shadwell and Egan.

III

It would obviously be wrong to see the two universities in the forty or so years before 1914 as consumed by the games cult, important as it was for many of the undergraduates. There were, as always, distinguished and notable scholars and not all students were pressurised into conformity. When M. R. James went to King's College, Cambridge, in 1882, he looked briefly at the river and then abandoned it for ever in favour of music and architecture. Nobody seems to have thought the worse of him for that.[43] Nor were games free from gentle and, on occasions, cruel ribaldry. During the early 1880s, the Cambridge University Boat Club was opposed to the granting of full blues for Rugby Union Football and the issue was debated at the Union. One undergraduate, Leo Maxse, noted for his total disinterest in games of any kind, decided to champion the cause of the Rugby players by constant reference in his speech to CUBC as the University Bicycle Club: 'He ploughed on, reiterating the words "Cambridge University Bicycle Club" with scathing contempt, till the tables were dissolved in laughter: the blue was granted, of course, in the end.'[44]

Like any large community of the young and the energetic, the universities were a compound of diverse interests and enthusiasms. J. E. Morgan, a former oar and physician, writing in 1873, listed what he saw as some of the alternatives to organised games: 'The strange innovations at the universities' he called them disapprovingly, 'ritualistic excesses; latitudinarian proclivities; socialistic crotchets; Darwinian theories of Simian descent; the dangerous intrustion of "sweet girl-graduates" at lectures and in common rooms.'[45] There was another he did not dwell on but one that L. R. Farnell, in time to become Rector of Exeter, Oxford, and Vice-Chancellor of the University, was acutely aware of. Not unsympathetic to the games-playing undergraduates, he nevertheless regretted the manner in which sporting activities encroached on matters academic 'by the withdrawal of scholars and exhibitioners from intellectual work' and he regretted 'the attempts of headmasters to influence our scholarship selections by athletic testimonials'.[46] It was this latter point that was crucial for, if one point of origin of the games cult was the oarsmen at the universities, it was quickly reinforced by a number of mid-Victorian public school headmasters such as Charles Vaughan at Harrow, Edward Thring at Uppingham and G. E. L. Cotton at Marlborough. Initially using organised games as an expedient to create some semblance of order and discipline, they allowed their successors and minions to turn them into a powerful and dominating force in many schools.

At the three main rowing schools of the first half of the century, Eton, Westminster and Shrewsbury, various headmasters had done their best to discourage any form of boating at all but, perhaps because it was a forbidden pleasure, it had managed to survive. At Eton and Westminster, one reason for its being frowned upon was the dangerous state of the Thames and its various bridges, a point made clear by one Eton parent towards the end of the eighteenth century: 'In respect to other masculine employments in the open air, I have no objection to rowing, provided it be accompanied with certain proper restrictions; for it never should be permitted at a public school, but under the inspection of some authorised person.'[47] Nevertheless, it was to continue, forcing headmasters into often equivocal positions. The first race between Eton and Westminster had taken place in 1829 and there was another in 1831, Dr Keate, the headmaster of Eton, apparently being kept in ignorance of it until the celebrations surrounding the victorious Etonians brought it to his attention: 'The sequel was a solemnly decorous lecture from the Doctor in "Keate's Chamber" to the eight. But the Doctor was evidently, nevertheless, well pleased.'[48] Headmasters of Westminster seem to have been placed in an equally uncertain position by the determination of the boys. In 1838 the Eton boat was ready to race when it was discovered that Westminster could not raise a full crew, the headmaster having used various ruses to detain some of those involved.[49] Ten years later, a different headmaster, Dr Liddell, refused leave for a challenge to be sent to Eton, reinforcing his prohibition in 1851 but, inconsistently, allowing a race against Oxford.[50] At Shrewsbury, Dr Kennedy threatened to take the local boatmen before the magistrates if they persisted in hiring out crafts to his pupils, but the boys then managed to acquire some of their own. The headmaster bowed to the inevitable and, in 1836, rowing was officially allowed – Eton doing the same four years later.[51] Nor, once Dr Liddell had departed to become Dean of Christ Church, Oxford, in 1855, were there any more contrary judgements from the headmaster's study at Westminster.[52]

By the second half of the century, rowing was recognised as an integral part of the games system at those schools where there was a reasonable river. Radley, Cheltenham, Derby Grammar School and Magdalen College School were among those that began to appear at Henley, while in the north, Durham School was prominent in the list of blues at Oxford and Cambridge. The supply of well-coached schoolboys to the two universities and colleges was in itself a powerful reinforcement not only to their standard of rowing but to the values that were becoming common both to the schools and to the undergraduates. Paradoxically, Dr Corrie, Master of Jesus College, Cambridge from 1874 to 1885, saw his college eight stay head of the river throughout his eleven year tenure in spite of his rooted belief that 'much evil was connected with rowing'. But he was virtually powerless in the face of the considerable interest taken in the boat club by two of his college officers, E. H. Morgan and H. A. Morgan.[53] Dr Cradock, while Principal of Brasenose College, Oxford, 1853–1886, was quite happy to encourage the acceptance of good oarsmen and cricketers without too much enquiry into their academic records.[54] Alfred Robinson, fellow of New College, Oxford, was taken to task by Sir Charles Oman for admitting too many Etonians. Nevertheless, they repaid Robinson handsomely enough since, between 1885 and 1906, the college was never out of the first three places in the Summer Eights and in 1897 won the Grand at Henley, equalling the course record.[55]

While there were dons willing to receive oarsmen and games-players in this manner, there was no shortage of headmasters and housemasters anxious to exploit the situation. Practically all of them were themselves former Oxford and Cambridge graduates, many in their youth having distinguished themselves on the games field or on the river. Probably the key element was the influence of certain kinds of housemasters who encouraged the emphasis on games and inspired boys in the belief that they were of prime importance in the life of the house and the school. Such was Edward Bowen at Harrow. 'I offer as my deliberate opinion', he once wrote,

> that the best boys are on the whole the players of games. I had rather regenerate England with the football elevens than the average Member of Parliament . . . When I reflect on the views to which games are a permanent corrective – laziness, foppery, man-of-the-worldness – I am not surprised at being led to the verdict which I have just delivered.[56]

It was the influence of men of this kind, the interest and enthusiasm that they showed, their degree of participation either as players or coaches, that was the final link in the reciprocal chain between the public schools and the universities. Just as some of the colleges accepted good games-players as students, so many headmasters were on the look out for athletic graduates for their staff, illustrated by the story of the undergraduate who, having scored a century in the university match at Lords, received telegrams offering him posts at five different schools.[57] The same happened with rowing. Men would leave the universities for the relative comfort of a public school common room and be totally content and satisfied coaching boys on the river. Such a one was H. M. Evans who went straight from University College, Oxford to Radley where, for thirty years from the late 1870s, he produced a succession of good, well-drilled crews.[58] By the eve of the Great War, Eton's reputation on the river was such that it attracted a number of men in a similar fashion.[59] They were not the first to take such an interest. Shadwell had been invited to look after the 1847 Eton eight and apparently produced a fine crew but the experiment was not repeated.[60] J. J. Hornby, a former Oxford rowing blue, who became first headmaster and then provost at Eton, might have seemed the archetypal athletic schoolmaster. In fact he rarely seems to have interested himself in such matters but what he did was to give his backing to the first man willing to take a serious and consistent interest in what the boys were doing on the water: the formidable Dr Edmond Warre.

Few men have dominated a sport in quite the manner adopted by Dr

Warre. His influence on several generations of schoolboys was to be profound and, through them, his tentacles reached to the universities. Adapting the methods of Shadwell and Egan – and, although he gave him no credit, those of Matthew Taylor who coached one of his Oxford crews – Warre laid down the firm principles of what was to become known as the English orthodox style of rowing, an approach that lasted until its watery grave when the Oxford crew sank in 1951.[61] As important, his own development of the values he had inherited from Shadwell and Egan were to take the elitist principle to the point of insular parochialism. A large, dominating man, he prompted one of his masters, A. C. Benson, to write of him that 'his eloquence is nil, his arguments unsound, his knowledge limited, his prejudices extreme, but yet, he is impressive in a high degree'.[62] His record, nevertheless, was impeccable. As an undergraduate at Balliol, he obtained firsts in both Classical Moderations and Greats and subsequently was elected a fellow of All Souls. In addition, he rowed in the 1857 and 1858 Boat Races, was president of OUBC and won a Henley medal. Though few boys would have dared to question his methods of coaching, Warre nevertheless was careful and scrupulous in his dealings with the schoolboy oarsmen, expecting to be invited each time the eight boated.[63] In theory he tried to keep rowing in proportion. Sir John Edwards-Moss, captain of boats in 1869, recalled that 'Warre's fixed principle was that school work, or any other duty, must come first, and rowing (or any other game) second'.[64] In practice these were probably pious hopes and boys set themselves to impress him. Occasionally, as happened to Guy Nickalls, some fault brought out all Warre's prejudices and forced the offending boy to unparalleled feats to gain his place in the boat.[65] And Warre had his limitations. Although an enthusiast in making experiments in both boat and oar design, his vision was impaired by the most important development of the 1870s, the sliding seat. It seems he never fully understood its use and would never allow any longer than eight inches.[66] His most accomplished successor as Eton coach, R. S. de Havilland, whom Warre had dropped from the school crew, felt that, towards the end of his coaching years, some of Warre's inspiration had gone. de Havilland once commented impatiently of his methods that 'to him style and the straight back became everything, and pace, or the winning of races, comparatively unimportant.'[67]

Whatever his faults, Warre by the sheer force of his considerable personality, exerted an influence that went far beyond Eton College. There had been resistance to his innovations. His presence on the

tow-path was at first seen as destroying the boys' 'charm of independence' and harming them by 'the emasculating influence of nursing'.[68]
When he first took the Eton eight to Henley and, above all, when it
recorded its first of many wins in the Ladies Challenge Plate in 1864, the
university oarsmen feared it would ruin the regatta, largely, as
Woodgate guessed, because men disliked being beaten by schoolboys.[69]
Such carping was quickly dissipated. At the 1866 Henley, of the twenty-
eight medals awarded for eights and fours, twenty-seven of them went
to nineteen Etonians, past and present, seventeen of them coached by
Warre.[70] The debt owed by the universities to Eton can be seen in the 281
from the school who rowed in the Boat Race between 1829 and 1929, just
over 40 per cent.[71] A significant number of them had been given their
first grounding at schools either by Warre or by de Havilland. It is
difficult not to believe that, as happened with Shadwell, Egan and
Stephen, they did more than just teach the rudiments of good rowing.
Others seemed to think so. Once, while coaching the eight, de Havill-
and noticed another master, known to have no interest in rowing,
watching and listening intently. When asked what he was doing, the
man confessed, 'I came down to hear the truth told.'[72]

A bond was being formed between the universities and the schools,
more particularly with Eton, that strengthened the existing exclusive
values of the Isis and the Cam. It was a potent reinforcement and one in
which there could be no questioning of the amateur status. It was
recognised in 1907 when the then president of OUBC, concerned that
the principles of good rowing should be maintained, decided to arrange
a number of lectures. It was almost inevitable that they should be given
by Edmond Warre and subsequently published as his final testament.[73]

IV

The emergence of the universities and the acknowledgement by some of
the schools that boating was an acceptable sport for schoolboys coincided with a radical transformation of rowing clubs in many parts of the
country. The crude *Iota* figures suggest that there was little organised
activity either on the Thames or elsewhere until the mid-1840s and even
then developments were to remain hesitant for some years to come. E.
D. Brickwood recalled that in 1852 'there was but little boat-racing
anywhere, the sport appearing temporarily on the wane'.[74] Two years
earlier there had been only fifteen entries at Henley and for a moment it
looked as if the regatta might not survive. In 1853 an Oxford spokesman

wrote to Cambridge suggesting a race at Henley 'which having already shown symptoms of decline, it was desirable by all means to endeavour to preserve'.[75] Leander, once so proud, seemed in danger of losing its way. In May 1855 an attempt to start the season by launching a new eight had to be abandoned in favour of boating only a four, the elements dissuading most of those present.[76] A year later, they could not even do that, only three being present and one of them declining to row, there 'being a Northeaster and having the snuffles.'[77]

The main causes of what Brickwood called 'this decadence of a manly and healthy sport – one so eminently British' were twofold. One was the state of the Thames and other rivers throughout the kingdom. Most of them were used as common sewers and, with increasing industrial waste, their state was both unpleasant and dangerous. To this, especially on the Thames, was added the increasing churning up of the water by barges and steamers, to the extent, according to Woodgate, that rowing 'was no longer the pleasant sport which it had been'.[78] But oarsmen were going to have to wait some years more before the quality of the Thames was improved, not until the London County Council, instituted in 1888, began to improve the whole drainage system of the City. The fact remains, nevertheless, that oarsmen had been prepared to risk possible dangers to their health from polluted waters for most of the early part of the century as long as there seemed some point and purpose to what they were doing.

But by the 1840s no clear pattern had emerged outside the university system and that of the professionals. There was a proliferation of small, unviable, often transitory clubs.[80] The problem was not confined to the Thames. In the North West, there had been a number of clubs that owned or used only one boat, manned by a group of friends. Such were the Red Rose at Lancaster, the Crusader at Liverpool and the True Bell at Chester.[81] At Durham Regatta, one event had been won in successive years, 1849 and 1850, by the Blue Bell and St Agnes, both probably being one-boat clubs and both quickly to disappear.[82] One reason why many of these clubs failed to survive was the high rate of the annual subscription and the fact that there was little margin for error if costs rose. In 1856, Leander's annual rate was five guineas, plus a guinea entrance fee for new members. But, in addition, its rules stated that 'if the yearly expenses exceed the annual subscriptions, they shall be borne rateably by those who were members at the time they were incurred'. Since at that time Leander's membership was limited to thirty-five, the additional costs were likely to be considerable.[83] For what were even smaller clubs, such as some of those in the North West and the North East, they were almost certainly terminal. Conditions were in fact against their survival at a time when, if a club had any pretensions at all, they would need to take advantage of the innovations in design and build of boats that were a feature of the 1850s.[84]

The *Iota* list gives some idea of how the more ambitious oarsmen began during these years to come to terms with some of these problems. Francis Playford of the old Thames Club was active from 1846 to 1849 on the water and, apart from successful forays to Henley, rested content with a limited reach of the river between Putney and Richmond. His younger brother, H. H. Playford, rowing during the 1850s, was more enterprising, being able to exploit the railways to travel further afield. In addition to all the normal Thames regattas, he was able to race as far afield as Manchester and Liverpool, often supported by two of his friends, Josias Nottidge and A. A. Casamajor.[85] They were all part of a small group of oarsmen who, using the Wandle Club and the Argonauts, were in the process of forming a centre of excellence on the Thames. Nevertheless, their aspirations seem to have run into exactly the same problems of costs as had ruined so many other small clubs. It was to find some solution to this state of affairs that Nottidge decided to summon a meeting on 9 April 1856 at the Craven Hotel in the Strand of 'gentlemen having at heart the interest of aquatic sports'.[86]

The discussions led directly to the setting up of London RC at Putney in the same year with the aim of offering a wide membership at a low subscription. By the end of May, 140 interested men had joined the new venture and by 1860 numbers stood at 194.[87] The cost was one guinea a year with an entry fee of the same amount.[88] Almost immediately the new club was a success. In June 1856 a letter was sent to Egan about the possibility of a match against the Oxford and Cambridge Subscription Rooms, though there is no record of any races having taken place, probably because the two university subscription clubs were moribund.[89] Initially London RC had to borrow equipment from Leander but by the beginning of the next year it was ordering new boats from Robert Jewitt on the Tyne. H. H. Playford was at pains to emphasise that the new club must have the best he could build: 'Just make these boats well and fast. We will put good men in them and they will then win their races which will be a great advertisement for you and then we shall see who will next get the most orders to build boats for London, Oxford and Cambridge. Your reputation is at stake. Mind what you do.'[90] Playford's confident cajolement was justified by the club's immediate successes at

Henley in 1857 when it won the Grand, the Stewards and the Diamonds.[91]

These victories were important in two ways. First, as Playford made clear in his letter to the boat-builder, London RC had every intention of establishing a standard at least as good as that of the universities and, secondly, its instant demonstration of good rowing highlighted the club's new structure and organisation. It was as a result the most influential of the large number of new clubs founded during the next twenty or so years. It was not, however, the first of its kind. Royal Chester had been founded on a similar basis in 1838, as had Henley RC the following year. It may be that these were premature experiments. The Chester Club's fortunes were so low by 1851 that it was in debt and had to auction the club's silver, although it had recovered magnificently by the middle of the decade with wins at Henley.[92] The crisis of mid-century had been of such a nature that it imperilled the majority of clubs but at least Chester and Henley RC had given some indication of the kind of organisation needed to ensure survival. Tyne Amateur Rowing Club had been set up in 1852 on much more modest lines than London RC in an attempt to solve what, if the *Iota* figures are to be believed, was a dearth in amateur rowing on that river. It seemed at first successful enough, 'upwards of sixty gentlemen immediately entered themselves as members'.[93] When, in November 1860, a meeting was held in Durham to consider founding a new club on the Wear, those present considered draft rules based on those of Tyne ARC and London RC. It was a prudent approach, taking heed of the particular problems of a near-neighbour as well as following the example of a highly successful metropolitan club.[94]

The London RC organisation was to be copied by a great many clubs, some new, others made up of smaller ones that decided to amalgamate. In nearly every case, however, accident, local conditions or other issues also played a part. Royal Chester's recovery owed much to its successes at Henley in 1855 and 1856, the latter year being particularly important since it won both the Grand and the Ladies in Matthew Taylor's new keelless eight. The fact that the crew could not apparently row the craft properly merely served to advertise both the type of boat and the club's considerable achievement.[95] In 1867, the old Lancaster RC collapsed, spawning in its place two new ones, the first of the same name, the second the John O'Gaunt Club. But this had less to do with any marked renewal of enthusiasm for rowing in the area than with fierce, partisan political differences dating from the 1865 election. One of the clubs became largely Tory in complexion, while John O'Gaunt sported the Liberal banner.[96] Nor were all new clubs originally founded to provide competitive rowing. The Grosvenor RC in Chester was set up in July 1869 to provide recreation for local clerks and shop assistants.[97] The more famous Thames RC had similar origins, founded in 1861 to give pleasure boating to the clerks and salesmen of the large London drapery warehouses and like institutions. By the 1870s, however, both its aims and composition were in the process of changing. W. H. Eyre, an early member, recalled that at the turn of the century there were 'very few (if any) "rag-trade" men in the club now. The social status (conventionally speaking) is, I suppose, higher.'[98] At its annual general meeting in 1884, the list of new members for election contained, apart from one clerk, men of eminently conventional backgrounds in the City of London, including merchants, insurance-brokers and a publisher. It seems obvious that, from modest and perfectly respectable beginnings, Thames RC was by the 1880s able to attract similar applicants to London RC while at the same time achieving comparable success on the water.[99] Leander, the only one of the old Thames-based clubs to survive, managed to revive its flagging fortunes almost by accident. It was never an open club like the others, but in an apparent attempt to control its membership, it introduced a university qualification which, paradoxically, made the club increasingly attractive to Oxford and Cambridge oarsmen. It took Leander some years to realise what a rich seam it could tap but, once it had done so, many of its best Henley crews were drawn from the two universities.[100]

The emergence of these new clubs gave some fresh vitality to rowing during the last thirty years of the century, paralleled by the reorganisation of regattas on many English rivers. Annual regattas, especially if professionals were involved, were always likely to attract spectators in some numbers. After the first Tyne Regatta in September 1834, one local newspaper commented that 'the surprise is that, with such facilities, the regatta should have been the first to be held upon the Tyne'.[101] Organisers, however, needed to be constantly on the alert if they were to hold the attention of the crowd and to attract the spectators back the next year. One press comment after the first Reading Regatta in 1842 was that there should be 'something to fill up the intervals between the races, which sometimes makes these entertainments dull and tedious affairs'.[102] Fouling and accusations of cheating, especially if professionals were present, could only add to the excitement as could races between those who did not normally exert themselves on rivers.

Watching people make fools of themselves has always had an appeal to some. Such was the fare offered at Worcester Regatta in 1845 with all kinds of odd aquatic games in addition to racing.[103] But the commercial element could have disagreeable results. A Lancaster RC crew clearly did not enjoy the Manchester and Salford Regatta in 1846, describing it as usual a blackguard, disreputable affair got up by a set of publicans and garden owners for their own particular benefit'.[104] But organisers were frequently faced with this kind of dilemma if they wanted to make their regattas successful. During the early 1860s, Derby Regatta had attracted a number of professional crews from Newcastle, Manchester and the Thames, Harry Clasper being one of the competitors. The crowds had been drawn by the presence of some of the best oarsmen in England. In 1863 the particular event was withdrawn and the regatta slumped, nobody being particularly interested in just watching amateurs competing against each other. It was an odd decision, not taken in any way to discourage professional rowing. It seems the local Derby watermen were upset at having no chance of winning against their more famous and talent rivals from other rivers. The result was that, after 1862, they were not able to race at all.[105]

The emergence of new clubs meant that many of them, as at Agecroft and at Evesham, started their own regattas so that by the 1880s a number of local circuits had been established. In other places, such as Durham, the setting up of a local rowing club breathed new life into an old regatta. Durham ARC began to take over the local regatta from its original founders, the university students, who became involved in a long-standing dispute over its date because of examinations.[106] An anonymous commentator congratulated the club on its efforts in 1863, certain that it 'will learn from experience how to perfect their arrangements in future. Durham is no doubt much indebted to them for taking the thing in hand.'[107] That the consequences of all this led to some lack of excitement and spontaneity seems to be the implied criticism of one newspaper after the turn of the century: 'Time was when Durham Regatta was a confusing jumble of aquatics and junketing. Those days are passed . . . The affair has naturally developed – and not recently either – from the haphazard methods of the early days to a systematic and business-like plane.'[108] Not all regattas, however, became quite so worthy and the emergence of new clubs did not always mean that old practices were forgotten in order to entertain the crowd. In 1884 and 1885, York had organised an aquatic festival, including, in addition to the normal rowing events, swimming handicaps, various non-rowing water contests such as a steeplechase over poles in the river, a tournament between scullers dressed as medieval knights that resulted in 'a great many upsets and ludicrous positions for the contestants and much laughter on the part of the spectators'.[109] By 1900 the Worcester committee also had a large number of additional events, among them a gymnastic display, costume and sack races, a cross-country event for the Volunteer Cyclist Corps, sword drill by a squad of Hussars and a marching and drill display by the Rifle Volunteers.[110]

All this suggests that, in the wake of the reconstruction of clubs from the 1850s onwards, there was a good deal of activity, much of it purposeful and rewarding. Private matches ceased to be the staple concern of amateur oarsmen apart from the Boat Race, one of the few remaining links with a less well organised and more rumbustious past. Of the new regattas, the best known was the Metropolitan, set up in 1866 under the aegis of London RC. It never quite fulfilled the hopes of its founders that it might rival Henley, largely because it never proved particularly attractive to the university and college crews.[111] Its relative failure highlighted the increasing importance of Henley Royal Regatta, as it was called after 1851 when Prince Albert became its patron. Its recovery from near extinction during the early 1850s has less to do with royal blessing than with it becoming the only place where the best of the new clubs, in the main those based on the metropolitan Thames, could compete on equal terms with the university-based oarsmen. London RC, Kingston RC and then Thames RC were establishing a standard of excellence that spurred each other on and, so Woodgate believed, forced the universities and the colleges to reassess their own standards.[112] The success of these clubs can be seen in Table V where the university monopoly before 1856 of the Grand and the Stewards, the two senior Henley events, was very effectively challenged up to the eve of the Great War.

The dominance of these Thames-based clubs gathered momentum during the rest of the nineteenth century but one consequence was that some of the smaller ones suffered, not least because they tended to act as feeders to the larger.[113] The result was to complete the process of closing a number of small and insubstantial clubs such as Ariel and Ilex and at the same time prevent others such as Corsair and Palmerston from establishing any kind of firm base.[114] Ariel, for example, recognising its difficult position, suggested to Thames RC in 1869 that it might amalgamate with its more vigorous neighbour, assuming the latter was prepared to pay £22 for their boats. Less than generously, the Thames RC committee offered only £12 and a waiving of the customary entrance

Table V *Comparison of winners – Grand and Stewards*

	Grand Challenge Cup			
	University and colleges	University and Club-based*	Thames-based	Provincial
To 1856	13	2	2	1
1857–1900	16	9	19	—
	Stewards Challenge Cup			
To 1856	10	2	3	1
1857–1900	18	3	22	1

Note: *Includes crews such as the Oxford Club of London, the Cambridge Subscription Rooms, and Leander which, though rowing as clubs, were largely manned by university undergraduates.

free.[115] Similar trends can be seen in the provinces. On the Tyne, for example, two active clubs, Ryton RC and Newcastle RC had both ceased to exist by 1914, the main beneficiary being the Tyne ARC and similar closures were to be found in the North-West.[116]

The most important development, however, had been the rise to prominence of a few metropolitan Thames clubs, the most active and influential being London RC. Not many provincial clubs saw themselves in the same league, the only exception being Royal Chester. Not only were these clubs setting high standards on the water but they completed a triumvirate of strength with the Isis and the Cam. Henley Royal Regatta became the focus of their attention, the only event where they could test their skills against each other. It was a mark of their acceptance that nobody ever raised any objections to the likes of London RC contesting the Henley trophies against the universities and colleges for, in the process or organising themselves, each of them had unhesitatingly accepted the unwritten rules of conduct and behaviour that had been at the heart of the ideas of Selwyn, Shadwell and Egan. In doing so they had become part of a powerful and dominant praetorian guard.

Notes

1 Neil Wigglesworth, *Rowing in the North West* (unpublished M.Ed. thesis, Manchester University, 1983), p. 44; A. A. Macfarlane-Grieve, *A History of Durham Rowing,* (Newcastle-on-Tyne, 1922), p. 17.
2 W. B. Woodgate, *Boating* (London, 1888), p. 192.
3 R. D. Burnell, *Henley Regatta – A History* (London, 1957), p. 43.
4 Macfarlane-Grieve, *A History of Durham Rowing*, pp. 34–6.

5 Burnell, *Henley Regatta*, p. 43.
6 W. J. Macmichael, *The Oxford and Cambridge Boat Races* (Cambridge, 1870), p. 77.
7 *Ibid*, pp. 78–9.
9 R. C. Lehmann, *The Complete Oarsman*, 1908 (London), pp. 4–5.
9 Cambridge University Boat Club was founded in 1829, the Oxford club not until ten years later.
10 W. E. Sherwood, *Oxford Rowing* (Oxford, 1900), p. 11.
11 G. C. Drinkwater and T. R. B. Saunders, *The University Boat Race: Official Centenary History* (London, 1929), p. 11.
12 Lehmann, *The Complete Oarsman*, p. 7. It is not at all clear how the amount of these wagers was in fact raised.
13 Macmichael, *Oxford and Cambridge*, pp. 53–7.
14 *Ibid.*, pp. 77–8.
15 In the Boat Race of December 1849, Oxford were awarded the race because an error by the Cambridge cox led to a foul. The secretary of CUBC wrote a letter regretting the incident since 'it very much disturbed the harmony and good feeling which should exist between the members of the rival universities in such contests.' (Macmichael, *Oxford and Cambridge* pp. 163–5). Although wager racing had ceased to exist as far as the university crews were concerned, there remained a number of sweepstakes at college level, Benjamin Jowett, the future Master of Balliol, being involved in one during the summer of 1837 (Geoffrey Faber, *Jowett – A Portrait with Background* (London, 1957, p. 115.) Sweepstakes for both sculling and punting continued at Eton until mid-century (L. S. R. Byrne and E. L. Churchill, *The Eton Book of the River* (Eton, 1935), p. 191).
16 Drinkwater and Saunders, *Boat Race*, p. 161.
17 W. W. Rouse Ball. *A History of First Trinity Boat Club* (Cambridge, 1908), p. 68.
18 Lehmann, *The Complete Oarsman*, pp. 16–17.
19 *Bell's Sporting Life in London*, 25 April, 1852. In 1875, Oxford temporarily broke their own rule, inviting Matthew Taylor, the boat-builder, to instruct the crew in the use of the new keelless boat (Lehmann, *The Complete Oarsman*, p. 16).
20 A. T. W. Shadwell, *Principles of Rowing* (London, 1846), p. 25. Originally published anonymously but now accepted as Shadwell's work (see F. Brittain, *Oar, Scull and Rudder – A Bibliography of Rowing* (London, 1930), p. 1).
21 Montague Sherman, *Athletics and Football* (London, 1889, third ed.), pp. 40–53.
22 W. Tuckwell, *Reminiscences of Oxford* (London, 1900), pp. 113–4.
23 W. B. Woodgate, *Reminiscences of an Old Sportsman* (London, 1909), pp. 365–87.
24 Mary Prior, *Fisher Row – Fishermen, Bargemen, and Canal Boatmen in Oxford, 1500–1900* (Oxford, 1982), p. 301.
25 Sherwood *Oxford Rowing* pp. 25–26 and 90–92; Prior, *Fisher Row*, p. 301.
26 Leslie Stephens, 'Athletics, sports and university studies', *Fraser's Magazine*, II, New Series, 1870, p. 694.
27 F. W. Maitland, *The Life and Letters of Leslie Stephen* (London, 1906), pp. 59–64.
28 Noel Annan, *Leslie Stephen* (London, 1951), p. 29; Maitland, *The Life and*

Letters p. 77; R. B. Martin, *The Dust of Combat: A Life of Charles Kingsley* (London, 1959), pp. 219–20.

29 S. Rothblatt, *The Revolution of the Dons: Cambridge and Society in Victorian England* (London, 1968), p. 171.

30 For further discussion of the cult of athleticism, see David Newsome, *Godliness and Good Learning* (London, 1961), Chapter IV; J. A. Mangan, *Athleticism in the Victorian and Edwardian Public Schools* (Cambridge, 1981), *passim*; H. R. Harrington, *Muscular Christinaity — A Study of a Victorian Idea* (Ph.D. thesis, Stanford University, 1971), *passim*; E. C. Mack and W. H. G. Armytage *Thomas Hughes*, (London, 1952), *passim*.

31 V. A. Hubur, quoted in M. M. Garland, *Cambridge Before Darwin* (Cambridge, 1980), pp. 2–3.

32 J. H. Newman, *The Idea of a University* (Oxford, 1976 ed.), Discourse VI, 9.

33 M. J. Wiener, *English Culture and the Decline of the Industrial Spirit* (Cambridge, 1982), pp. 22–4 and Oliver MacDonagh, *Early Victorian Government* (London, 1977), pp. 212–3.

34 Rothblatt, *The Revolution of the Dons*, pp. 86–7.

35 J. R. de S. Honey, *Tom Brown's Universe – The Development of the Victorian Public School* (London, 1977), *passim*.

36 V. H. H. Green, *Oxford Common Room – A Study of Lincoln College and Mark Pattison* (London, 1957), p. 260.

37 Maitland, *The Life and Letters*, p. 69.

38 V. H. H. Green, *The Commonwealth of Lincoln College, 1427–1977* (Oxford, 1979), pp. 415–6.

39 Maitland, *The Life and Letters* pp. 58–9. The Trinity Hall boat went Head of the River for the first time in the Lent term 1859. The college's greatest achievement was at the 1887 Henley when it won the Grand, the Ladies Plate, the Thames Cup, the Stewards and the Visitors.

40 *Ibid.*, pp. 48–9. The extract is from an anonymous article on rowing in Anthony Trollope, ed., *British Sports and Pastimes* (London, 1868). Maitland argues that he is certain Stephen was the author.

41 Rothblatt, *The Revolution of the Dons*, p. 228.

42 *Ibid.*

43 M. R. James, *Eton and King's – Recollections, Mostly Trivial* (London, 1926), pp. 143–4.

44 *Ibid*, pp. 162–3.

45 J. E. Morgan, *University Oars* (London, 1873), pp. 70–1.

46 L. R. Farnell, *An Oxonian Looks Back* (London, 1934), pp. 141–2.

47 L. S. R. Byrne and E. L. Churchill, *The Eton Book of the River* (Eton, 1935), p. 120.

48 Anonymous, *Rowing at Westminster from 1813 to 1883* (London, 1980), p. 23.

49 *Ibid.*, p. 47.

50 *Ibid.*, p. 71.

51 Byrne and Churchill, *The Eton Book*, p. 123.

52 *Ibid.*, pp. 122–3. In 1884 Westminster rowing temporarily stopped because of timetable difficulties.

53 A. Gray and Fr., Brittain, *A History of Jesus College, Cambridge* (London, 1960), pp. 171–3.

54 Honey, *Tom Brown's Universe*, p. 111.
55 J. Buxton and P. Williams, eds., *New College Oxford 1879–1979* (Oxford, 1979), pp. 98–9.
56 Mangan, *Athleticism*, pp. 154–161.
57 Honey, *Tom Brown's Universe*, p. 43.
58 L. Cecil Smith, *Annals of Public School Rowing* (Oxford, 1920), p. 23.
59 Byrne and Churchill, *The Eton Book*, pp. 214–5, 218.
60 *Ibid.*, p. 200.
61 P. Haig-Thomas and M. A. Nicholson, *The English Style of Rowing* (London, 1958), *passim*.
62 David Newsome, ed., *Edwardian Excursions – From the Diaries of A. C. Benson, 1898–1904* (London, 1981), p. 97.
63 C. R. L. Fletcher, *Life of Edmond Warre* (London, 1922), p. 272.
64 *Ibid.*, p. 281.
65 Guy Nickalls, *Life's A Pudding, An Autobiography* (London, 1939), pp. 50–7.
66 G. C. Bourne, *Memories of an Eton Wet-Bob of the Seventies* (London, 1933), pp. 90–1, 95–7; Byrne and Churchill, *The Eton Book*, p. 215.
67 Fletcher, *Life of Edmond Warre*, p. 278.
68 *Ibid*, p. 274.
69 Woodgate, *Boating* p. 209.
70 Byrne and Churchill, *The Eton Book* pp. 208–9.
71 E. Halladay, 'Of pride and prejudice: the amateur question in English nineteenth century rowing', *International Journal of the History of Sport*, vol 4, no. 1, May 1987.
72 Byrne and Churchill, *The Eton Book*, pp. 219–220.
73 Edmond Warre, *On the Grammar of Rowing* (Oxford, 1909), *passim*.
74 E. D. Brickwood, *Boat-Racing: Or the Arts of Rowing and Training* (London, 1876), p. 174.
75 Burnell, *Henley Regatta*, pp. 79–85.
76 *Bell's Life*, 6 May 1855.
77 *Leander Log*, 30 May 1856.
78 Woodgate, *Boating*, pp. 181–2.
79 Byrne and Churchill, *The Eton Book*, p. 13.
80 London RC, *From Strength to Strength – 1856–1981 – Portrait of London RC* (London, 1981), pp. 182–3.
81 Wigglesworth, *Rowing* (M.Ed. thesis), p. 49.
82 Macfarlane-Grieve, *A History of Durham Rowing*, p. 197.
83 Leander Log, *Rules*, 1856.
84 Two innovations were particularly important, the outrigger and the keelless boat. See Appendix I.
85 *Iota*, pp. 18–9, 75–6, 82–4.
86 London RC, *Strength to Strength*, p. 57.
87 *Ibid, p. 7*; London RC, *Letter Book and Accounts, 1859–60*.
88 London RC, *Letter Book*, 17 November, 15 December 1856.
89 *Ibid.*, 23 June 1856.
90 *Ibid.*, 28 June 1856, 13 February 1857.
91 Henley rules then as now prevent a club competing within a year of its foundation. In 1856 London RC entered under Argonaut colours, winning

the Stewards, Wyfolds, Goblets and Diamonds.

92 Keith Osborne, 'Royal Chester – the oldest open rowing club', *The Almanack*, 1988, pp. 230–4.

93 *Newcastle Daily Chronicle*, 17 December 1852.

94 *Durham Country Advertiser*, 23 November 1860.

95 Osborne, *The Almanack*, p. 232; Burnell, *Henley Regatta*, p. 86.

96 N. Wigglesworth, 'A history of rowing in the North West of England', *British Journal of Sports History*, 3, 1986.

97 *Ibid*.

98 W. H. Eyre, 'Thames Rowing Club' in Lehmann, *The Complete Oarsman*, pp. 179–205.

99 Thames RC, *Minutes*. 15 March 1884; London RC, *Letter Book – Memoranda*, dated November and December 1872.

100 R. D. Burnell and H. R. N. Rickett, *A Short History of Leander Club* (Henley, 1968), p. 17.

101 *Newcastle Journal*, 20 September 1834.

102 John Allen, 'Reading Regattas', *The Almanack*, 1965, pp. 192–6.

103 R. J. Davis, *Boating at Worcester in the Nineteenth Century* (Worcester, undated), p. 5.

104 N. Wigglesworth, *A Short History of Rowing in Lancaster*, typescript, ARA headquarters, p. 5.

105 J. Gretton, *et alia; Derwent Rowing Club – Centenary 1857–1957* (Derby, 1957), pp. 7–8.

106 Macfarlane–Grieve, *A History of Durham Rowing*, pp. 47, 67.

107 *Ibid*, pp. 38–9, 60–7.

108 *Durham County Advertiser*, 28 June 1907.

109 *York Herald*, 1 August 1885.

110 Davis, *Boating at Worcester*, p. 29.

111 Woodgate, *Boating*, pp. 42–3.

112 *Ibid*, p. 182.

113 R.P.P. Rowe and C. M. Pitman, *Rowing* (London, 1898), p. 185.

114 London RC, *Letter Book*, 9 May 1860 and Amateur Rowing Association, *List of Affiliated Clubs* 1913.

115 Thames RC, *Minutes*, 3, 11 February 1869.

116 Wigglesworth, Rowing in the North West, (M.Ed. thesis), p. 75.

3

Defining an amateur

The emergence of a coherent group of oarsmen and clubs during the late 1850s and 1860s, organised on similar lines and sharing similar values, was the most significant development that had to that time taken place in amateur rowing. Its effects were quickly felt. Henley Royal Regatta began to prosper and the stewards who organised it began to find themselves pushed into greater prominence by being forced to take decisions about which they at first showed some hesistancy and reluctance. London RC, the strongest of the metropolitan clubs, also found itself thrust into a position which demanded considerable initiative but which it was prepared to shoulder with some courage and sense of responsibility.

By the 1870s a good many of these Thames-based oarsmen were becoming aware that a number of problems had to be faced. Fundamental to them all was the need to come to grips with the issue of amateurism. The search for an adequate definition was to be long, arduous and frequently disagreeable. Those who formed the elite group, largely from the Thames and the two universities, were able to approach the problem with a degree of confidence. They possessed a coherent philosophy that had its roots in the universities and a set of values combining in equal measure those of the enterprising middle class and those of the older rural gentry, a pattern of life unique to this country. At first sight they seemed an immutable group, exclusive and class-conscious in outlook. In practice they were to prove more sensitive and accommodating than might have been expected. Certain of their own approach, they were able to make concessions that were important, particularly by coming to terms with the problems posed by foreign competitors, anxious to row in this country and in particular at Henley. It was to prove a declicate matter, not least since the social backgrounds of many overseas oarsmen were unlikely to mirror very closely those to be found in this country. The need to come to terms with foreign crews eager to test themselves against the best in England was to have a decisive effect on resolving the amateur issue, the crucial question during the last quarter of the century in English rowing.

I

The resolution of this major issue was to be the concern in the main of the leading metropolitan clubs and the Henley stewards. It is difficult to gauge precisely how much impact the question had on the smaller clubs, particularly those in the provinces. Few of them had any pretensions and, in spite of the opportunities offered by the railways, they remained largely parochial in outlook. Yet imperceptibly they began to accept similar values to those of the better-known clubs. Sometimes the influence of university men, clergymen and lawyers being the most obvious, set an example. But of equal importance was the need for a rowing club to be accepted locally and this often demanded certain standards of conduct. Nottingham RC's decision in 1862 to abandon its watermen members was taken after consulting the rowing editor of *Bell's Life*, none other than T. S. Egan, as well as after corresponding with London RC and, interestingly, Clydesdale RC. But it is clear that local insinuations, that the club might be embarking on the wrong course of action, had begun the process.[1] The need to be sensitive to what others might say, especially if it was a fledgling club, was to prove important.

In 1850 there were two less well-known boat races between the two universities, one at Cambridge in July and another at Oxford just over a month later. Neither was to figure in accounts of the University Boat Race since they were not between undergraduates but between the university and college servants. After the second race a dinner was held and one of the Cambridge crew declared that in spite of two defeats: 'they had met to contend for superiority in a manly sport and though Cambridge would return as losers, they felt not the slightest mortification, because they had been outweighed by the generous and noble spirits in which they had been received by all parties at Oxford'.[2] Shadwell and Egan could not but have applauded such sentiments.

Being based on the Isis and Cam, it was not surprising that such clubs absorbed as a matter of course the opinions of the undergraduates. Others followed suit. In 1889 the Reverend B. J. Kidd founded a rowing club at Oxford for his church, St Philip and St James, for young men resident in the parish or educated at the church school. Kidd was apparently much influenced by attitudes he found at Keble College, seeing the new club as a means of helping the less fortunate among his parishioners. There was a reading room, a small library and a billiard table for the winter months, together with a collection of boats for use during the summer. As the rowing side of the club developed, St John's College, the patrons of the living, allowed its members to use the college barge during the long vacation. St Philip and St James responded with impeccable behaviour, that reflected the attitudes of its founders and mirrored those of the college clubs that dominated the Isis. A former captain said of Kidd and of those who had helped him, that 'to them we owe the spirit of sportsmanship and good feeling which has become a tradition in the Club, and that loyalty and obedience to officers without which no club can have a prolonged existence'.[3]

It was perhaps not surprising that opinions of this nature should be found among the local town clubs at Oxford and Cambridge. But they were also echoed elsewhere suggesting that they were not the sole monopoly of the elite oarsmen. The founders of Durham ARC in 1860 took it as axiomatic 'that outdoor amusements and in the van cricket and boating are the very best means of bringing out the bone and muscle of our English youth'.[4] Such eminently proper sentiments were to be reinforced by Ishmael Lythgoe, in large measure responsible for setting up Agecroft RC on the Irwell in the same year as Durham, but in his case he added a strongly patriotic note as well. He was

> confident that no apology is necessary for such a proceeding when the physical as well as national advantages resulting from a love of aquatics is taken into consideration; for rowing has long held a very high position in the list of manly exercises and physical recreations, and, doubtless, has been a most essential element in the education of the bravest and ablest defenders of our country, to whose naval exploits England is mainly indebted for the high position it now holds amongst nations.[5]

Such grandiose sentiments seem, at first sight, at variance with the humble and often fragile beginnings of many of these clubs. Agecroft, for example, was forced during its difficult early years to store its original second-hand boat in an old boiler-house, while Derby RC, founded in 1879, rented two bridge arches from the Great Northern Railway.[6] Yet, in spite of their proverty, great emphasis seems to have been placed on the need to present a respectable appearance to the outside world. In 1883, Derby's officials, like those in many other clubs, insisted that the sabbath rule be strictly enforced and expelled a member for rowing on a

Sunday.[7] At the inter-collegiate regatta of the Oxford servants in 1882, the New College four included a professional oarsman. Great offence was taken and all but one of the other entries withdrew.[8] In June 1885, the committee of Durham ARC had no doubt that the behaviour of two of its oarsmen at Durham Regatta had broken the accepted code of practice while racing. It was agreed that they should be expelled unless they wrote letters approved by the committee to Middlesbrough Amateur Boating Club.[9]

Striking correct attitudes was not necessarily the consequence of received wisdom from those acquainted with standards and behaviour elsewhere. In some cases, no doubt, it was. Durham ARC during the last quarter of the century had six former Oxford and Cambridge blues among its members, several of whom were active on the water or as members of the committee and one of whom was a canon of the cathedral.[10] Agecroft, during the 1870s, benefited from the presence in the neighbourhood of two Cambridge blues, the brothers John and James Close.[11] But just as strong an influence was the realisation by club officials that good behaviour, on and off the water, was a matter of necessity. It was in the interest of these clubs not to offend the sensibilities of the community among which they lived. Both Durham ARC and Durham Regatta needed the goodwill of three important bodies in the city, the council, the dean and chapter and the university authorities, not least because between them they owned most of the riparian rights. The club's original boat-house stood on land leased from the university, while tentative plans to build another involved careful negotiations with the cathedral chapter.[12] Nor could a club or regatta afford to offend often powerful local dignatories who could on occasions be generous. In Durham, the Wharton family's bequest had included one of the two most important trophies for the regatta.[13] The same was true elsewhere. Evesham RC was indebted to the Rudge family, local landed gentry, which provided three successive presidents for the club. The first of them, E. C. Rudge, bought the club a new boat in 1863 and continued to give generous subscriptions until his death.[14] Occasionally such deference to the great and the important could go sadly wrong and be the cause of some embarrassment. In 1909, the committee of the Tyne ARC discovered that a former treasurer could not account for a financial gift from the Duke of Northumberland. It was an unfortunate business that was never properly explained.[15]

The standing of a club or regatta in the eyes of the local community was important and it imposed its own obligations. The establishment of cordial relations might mean the possibility of assistance and certainly the acceptance of rowing as part of the character of a place, adding something to the pleasure and quality of life. Evesham RC was able fairly early to establish itself in this way. It originally combined its regatta with the annual horticultural show and by 1869 seemed firmly fixed in the public's favour. The *Evesham Journal* reported that 'the fete, picnic, and flower-show were held on the workman Pleasure Grounds and also on the playing fields opposite, both of which are capital situations for the purpose, being close to the centre of the town and having at their foot, gliding like time, unresting and unhastening, the soft-flowing Avon'. There was an enclosure on one side of the river, where 'the cream of the counties disported themselves . . . and the proletariat flocked to the Fleece Meadow opposite, where all the fun of the fair was in progress'. It was clearly a popular occasion even though, in later years, the officials could only afford the band of the local militia rather than that of the Coldstream Guards.[16] During the years before 1914, Evesham RC exploited its good standing in the town, offering pleasure boating, tennis, the use of a gymnasium as well as a reading room. At a time when, except at the universities, rowing was normally a summer sport, some of these facilities would remain open during the winter months at a reduced subscription.[17] Alert to all possibilities, the club's committee was prepared in 1913 to accept the services of the new picture-house in the town, allowing the screening of scenes from the regatta as long as the owner paid the proper price.[18]

Evesham's efforts to diversify and to offer the services of the club to as wide a cross-section of the public as possible went rather further than most. But many clubs recognised that not everybody was interested in competitive rowing and that a significant number simply wanted to use boats for pleasure. Boating, as distinct from rowing, had in fact the longer pedigree. It had been common enough on most English rivers for many years and by the middle of the century travellers were beginning to explore the waterways of the continent.[19] There were obvious commercial possibilities in all this and by the 1870s and 1880s few parts of the country were without boating facilities of some kind. Jerome K. Jerome's *Three Men in a Boat*, published in 1889, highlighted the delights of this relaxed approach, as did Charles Dickens, junior's, *Dictionary of the Thames*.[20] *The Almanack* was responding to such needs by the 1870s, providing guides, advice and information, while its advertisers, often boat-building and riverside hoteliers, all underlined the availability of boats for hire.[21] Such ventures, as at Hollingworth Lake, near Rochdale, sometimes spawned their own rowing clubs, parallel with the pleasure boating enterprise.[22] A great many clubs tried to cater for this need. Thames RC basically owed its origins to this form of rowing as did, among others, Runcorn RC in the North-West, while even the highly competitive London RC tried to satisfy those who simply wished to boat for pleasure.[23] At the Stratford-upon-Avon club women were admitted as members simply to use the pleasure boats and the systems seemed to work well enough apart from the nuisance caused by those, not always female, who could not manage the punts.[24] But in any case, much of the early rowing in many of the clubs was of a far from serious nature. Although occasionally sending a four to race at the Agecroft Regatta, Hollingworth Lake's main efforts were at first devoted to organising internal club races, usually of scratch crews, a pattern that was to be found among many rowing clubs. Although no doubt giving a great deal of pleasure, skill seems to have been at a premium.[25]

Inevitably the presence in one club of members with different aims and aspirations could create tension. At Worcester RC, the arguments led in 1878 to a temporary closure, the revived club resolving that: 'for the present the club should be for competitive rowing only'. But such determination did not end the disagreements since, if it was to survive, the club needed as wide a membership as possible.[26] That in its turn, however, inevitably meant some extra expenditure on suitable types of boats. By 1901, for example, Exeter Amateur Rowing Club had, in addition to its five fours, seven skiffs and a tub pair, five dinghies for pleasure boating, a canoe and a punt.[27] Tees Amateur Boating Club, though on a far from salubrious river and aware of the need to limit its costs, still felt it was worth investing in two new pleasure boats in 1922 in an attempt to widen its appeal.[28] In the end, very often for financial reasons, the competitive element in a club triumphed, though not always without some bitter argument. In 1937 Stratford-upon-Avon RC decided to sell all boats not needed for racing and training but it was a decision made only after a particularly tense debate.[29]

Assuming club officials were able to reconcile different needs, the advantages of allowing members a choice of activities were obvious. Evesham RC, for example, was particularly successful in this way and by 1898 its membership stood at 105, a healthy number compared with Durham ARC which largely confined its efforts to competitive rowing. In 1890 it had twenty-seven ordinary and eight honorary members with £1 15s in the bank. 'Every effort should be made to increase our number of members with a view to raising the needful funds', wrote the pessimistic secretary.[30] Twelve years later he could still describe the numbers in the club as meagre 'and were it not for the advent of five officers from the Newcastle Barracks, our fighting members would be small indeed'.[31] Nevertheless, whether viable or not, clubs of this kind made rowing an acceptable part of the local scene during the latter years of the century. They generated their own set of values and imposed their own codes of behaviour as much through necessity as through precept. They dared not offend otherwise they would lose much public goodwill. There was little money in amateur rowing and yet the costs of equipment were considerable. Even when charges to the public were allowed for entry to a regatta, the finances always needed additional subsidies. At Durham, the regatta committee appointed a number of local collectors who, dividing the city between them, solicited subscriptions from businessmen and householders. It was a mark of the esteem in which the regatta was held and, by implication, the local rowing club, that such a system did not appear to have caused resentment.[32]

This sense of being a part of the local community was probably more important in setting the tone of a club or a regatta than anything else. If a university or college oarsman took an interest, he simply gave his seal of approval to a code of values that was unlikely to differ much from his own. The opportunity offered by the local regatta was, therefore, all the more important. It was the only public demonstration in the year of the virtues of the sport and if additional but respectable entertainments were available as well, so much the better for the club concerned in the organisation. The cachet was the greater if well-known crews from outside the area could be attracted, all the more so if they came from one of the universities or from the metropolitan Thames. The winning of the Grand at Durham in 1857 by a four from Lady Margaret, Cambridge, was greeted with considerable pleasure and approval.[33] At Oxford, the local clubs had their own separate pattern of rowing from that of the college crews and one of the main events of the season was the Oxford Royal Regatta. Nobody objected in 1875 when a scratch crew of undergraduates, resident during the vacation, entered for the main event as the Oxford Vacation Club. The eight was a good one, containing two future blues as well as J. Lowndes, five times winner of the Diamonds at Henley and twice holder of the Wingfield Sculls. It won the event with some ease and four similar crews were to do the same up to 1885. F. J. Vincent of the Falcon RC at Oxford had no doubt that their presence at the regatta did much to further its enjoyment and its success.[34]

There is an obvious note of deference in Vincent's gratitude towards undergraduate patronage of the local regatta. When circumstances were reversed, however, the reaction could be less than generous. As early as 1846, Lancaster Regatta took the advice of *Bell's Life* about the advisability of admitting a crew of tradesmen to an event intended for amateurs. The reply was full of the need for careful and subtle social distinctions, stating that:

> on the London river many members of the most distinguished amateur clubs are engaged in trade. This does not include journeymen or mechanics whose crews are usually called "landsmen" to distinguish them from gentlemen amateurs and professional watermen. If the oarsmen in question are master tradesmen, the decision should stand; if journeymen or mechanics, they should be defaulted.[35]

But, as E. D. Brickwood realised twenty years later, clubs had not always shown such careful discrimination in the way they selected their members, nor were there any guide-lines for them to follow assuming they wished to.[36] Nor were regatta authorities always prepared to make the kind of difficult judgements that would seek to distinguish between the social status or the type of work of competitors. When, however, they did, the confusion and the disagreements could be uncomfortable. At Agecroft Regatta in 1874, clubs from as far distant as the Thames, the Tyne and the Cam had been persuaded to attend. It was a minor triumph for a small north-western club and may well have been a tribute to the influence of the Close brothers. But another entry was from the Bolton and Ringley Club which, having won its event, was suddenly disqualified. The arguments were prominently discussed in the local press where the Agecroft secretary justified his decision on the grounds that the Bolton men were artisans. In replying, the Bolton Club raised in measured tones what was to be the crucial issue:

> If any gentlemen would kindly give us a true definition of what an amateur is, we should feel greatly obliged, as we have always been under the impression that if a person did anything for pleasure and not for money, that person was an amateur, but if he should do anything for money, or in any shape for his living, he loses his title to be an amateur.[37]

II

The dilemma was that no authority existed to answer such a question. Although the problems raised by overseas entries were soon to force the Henley stewards to face such issues, they never showed any inclination to don the kind of mantle worn by the Royal and Ancient Golf Club or the Marylebone Cricket Club. The only alternative was the opinion of well-known individuals. T. S. Egan, especially in his capacity as a writer for *Bell's Life*, was the most influential. Another was the rowing correspondent of *The Field*, E. D. Brickwood, a winner of both the Diamonds at Henley and the Wingfield Sculls. Middlesbrough ABC consulted both in 1877 as to whether or not the club should return a trophy to the defunct Roundhay Park Regatta at Leeds, ignoring the views of both that they would be wrong to keep the cup.[38] It was hardly a satisfactory way of settling matters, especially as the views of particular individuals would not necessarily always command universal respect.

The problem was likely to be greater if the issues discussed were largely those of principle. During the 1850s and 1860s, the question of the exact meaning of amateurism began to loom larger in the minds of some oarsmen and it was Brickwood who put forward a definition, in 1866, whose nature suggests that already some of the clubs and regattas were thinking on somewhat narrow and socially exclusive lines, very different from the relaxed approach of men like Woodgate. Brickwood hoped that his views would

> perhaps suffice for all ordinary purposes – Amateurs must be officers of Her Majesty's Army, Navy or Civil Service, members of the Clerical, Medical or Legal professions, of the Universities of Oxford, Cambridge, Dublin, London, Durham, Edinburgh, Glasgow, St. Andrew's or Aberdeen, and the Queen's Colleges in Ireland, of Eton, Radley, Westminster and other public schools, or of any established club not composed of tradesmen or working mechanics, which would be allowed by the stewards of the Henley-on-Thames Regatta to compete for their Grand Challenge Cup, Stewards Cup, Silver Goblets or Diamond Sculls.[39]

There can be little doubt that Brickwood's lone enterprise reflected the views of a good many at that time and it may well be that the secretary at Agecroft in 1874 had this definition in mind when he disqualified the Bolton and Ringley crew.

However it was used, it remains a revealing summary, not least because Brickwood takes acceptance at Henley as one of the touchstones of amateurism. But what is equally interesting is what he leaves out. There is no mention at all of not rowing against a professional, nor does his definition prevent an amateur competing for a money prize. In fact Brickwood had no objection to the latter; just the opposite. He regretted the decision in 1861 to abolish the Wingfields as a sweepstake and stated that he was 'not disposed to consider that the bare fact of contending for a prize within the United Kingdom, either wholly or in part money, deprives a gentleman of his right to be considered an amateur'.[40] Possibly some of the Henley stewards shared his point of view since in 1866 they saw no reason for disqualifying Woodgate after he had raced a professional sculler for a one-sided bet from Putney to Hammersmith.[41] Nevertheless such a line of thinking was not in accord with the firm ideas that were becoming holy writ on the Isis and the Cam, however much some of their representatives, such as Woodgate, might try to suggest otherwise. It is difficult to believe that someone like Egan would have seen Brickwood's definition as anything other than inadequate.

There was, therefore, some degree of confusion. By the third quarter of the century, the robust attitudes of an earlier age were in part being questioned but there was nobody with any real authority to act as a guide to the bewildered. The reliance on the opinions of individuals meant that clubs and regattas could pick and choose at will, assuming they were aware of them. Part of the complaint of the Bolton and Ringley crew in 1874 had been their bafflement at the view of the Agecroft officials since they had been accepted elsewhere without anyone complaining of their presence.[42] The only way out of such a dilemma would be to find some kind of authoritative voice which others would be prepared to respect.

In fact such a body had only recently ceased to exist, although its influence was confined in the main to the Thames. It had been the apparent slump in rowing activity, during the late 1840s and early 1850s, that had prompted a number of oarsmen to consider some means of rescuing the sport. They produced a number of ideas but their most notable achievement was the setting up of London RC in 1856. Two years earlier, the prime mover in the group, Josias Nottidge, had founded the Thames National Regatta. His chosen instrument was the Thames Subscription Club, a purely advisory body, described in *The Almanack* of 1862 as existing 'to aid poor watermen and to encourage and foster rowing generally'.[43] Nottidge's original aim had been to use the Subscription Club as a source of ideas and as a means of raising sufficient funds to establish and support new regattas.[44] It was a measure of the strength of professional rowing at the time and of the continued interest in its progress by the leading amateurs that the only regatta that was established was a revival of the old Royal Thames Regatta, moribund since 1849. It may have been something of a disappointment to Nottidge and his associates that they failed to attract any amateur interest in the regatta until 1866, when the Subscription Club was in the process of winding-up its affairs. But it was also the date of the foundation of the Metropolitan Regatta, a purely amateur event, and by that time too, London RC was sufficiently strong to have absorbed most of the energy of Nottidge and his friends.[45]

While it lasted, however, the Thames National Regatta was a success but, more important, through its controlling body, the Subscription Club, attracted several influential amateurs, including A. A. Casamajor and T. S. Egan.[46] That, under this double umbrella, Nottidge managed to assemble a group of like-minded amateurs was important in itself. Certainly they saw themselves as having an influential role. Perhaps a little ingenuously, given the rowing editor's interests in its activities, *Bell's Life* could describe the Thames Subscription Club as 'representative of all rowing in England'.[47] It was a somewhat bold plea since it was not a governing body and never claimed to be. In the end its members channelled their energies into London RC, concluding presumably that the prerequisite for more vigorous amateur rowing was a more sensible club structure. But Nottidge and his group had left to London RC an important legacy. They had strongly hinted that all rowing – and in their case they included the professionals – needed an effective form of organisation. It was a responsibility that London RC was already prepared to accept.

At first its officials were mainly interested in establishing the new club on a sound basis but its immediate success, both in terms of recruitment and in the number of its victories at Henley, allowed its committee to consider other aspects of rowing. In 1859, for example, continuing the tradition of amateur patronage and reinforcing the initiative of the Thames Subscription Club, it instituted an annual race for a coat, badge and freedom among watermen's apprentices.[48] More important for the future of amateur rowing, London RC looked with some alarm at the continuance of a number of small clubs along the Thames, few of them apparently strong enough to survive for any length of time. Casamajor, listing in 1860 what he thought were the main boat clubs in the country, went on to mention some of the less strong such as Ariel, Corsair and Palmerston, each with a membership of between ten and twelve.[49] London RC, picking up one of Nottidge's notions of the early 1850s, put forward the idea that the best Thames-based oarsmen should amalgamate to produce stronger crews to compete at Henley. It envisaged for itself a gubernatorial role. At its annual meeting in 1861, the committee saw the club assuming the same position among the smaller clubs as the two university boat clubs had among the colleges. 'The London R.C. was the university crew of London' was the bold claim of a motion that was unanimously passed.[50] A first attempt to arrange matters in 1864 resulted, according to *The Sportsman*, in a 'disastrous fiasco'.[51] The next year, H. H. Playford of London RC continued the efforts, advancing the idea of amalgamated crews at a meeting on 9 February. It seems clear that the smaller clubs were suspicious of such an initiative and there was a considerable degree of resistance. By the final meeting on 4 August, all that was being discussed were arrangements for a procession of boats, races in eights and pairs and a dinner. By 1866 those somewhat timid conclusions had been translated into something a little more ambitious, the Metropolitan Regatta.[52]

For the first time, one influential club had tried to give some kind of lead and to encourage a reasonably cohesive approach. That the attempt was basically a failure was less important than the fact of its having been tried. As it was, London RC's involvement with the Metropolitan Regatta was to reinforce still further its view that some form of controlling body was needed, at least as far as the affairs of the metropolitan Thames were concerned. It already had some experience of the often unsatisfactory way that regattas could be conducted. In 1858, London found itself in dispute with Kingston RC over an incident at the latter's regatta and it blamed the local organisers for 'introducing into their regulations certain rules opposed, in the opinion of London R.C., to common sense'.[53] But it was to find its patience tested to the limit by some of the problems posed by the Metropolitan Regatta.

Although by far the strongest club on the committee, London RC, nevertheless, found that it was forced by the other representatives to accept demands that constantly compromised its own particular notions of how a regatta should be conducted.[54] The irritation at this state of affairs was further exacerbated by the increasing financial drain on London's resources due to the regatta's continual and growing deficit. The auditor's report of 1872 commented on the number of clubs that had not paid their subscriptions for several years and the same point was to be made again in 1876, 1879 and 1882, culminating in the secretary's statement on the 1884 regatta, that 'from a financial point of view it had been the most disastrous one we have had'.[55] For London RC this was an unacceptable state of affairs, one that raised doubts about what other whims and vagaries might exist elsewhere.

There was, however, another area that was to cause London RC concern, one that was to focus particular and immediate attention on the issue of amateurism. As early as 1860, the club's officials had tried to extend their horizons by proposing an international regatta at Putney.

Letters had been sent to 'gentlemen amateurs' as far afield as the United States, Sweden and Russia, as well as to France and to Belgium. It had been a disappointment when nothing had come of the project.[56] Nevertheless, it had entertained a number of American and German challenge matches on the Thames during the late 1860s and the 1870s, and it had been among the first clubs from this country to race abroad. On the whole, these latter ventures overseas had not been particularly happy experiences. At the 1867 Paris Exhibition Regatta, London RC had objected to a Canadian four, not because they rowed in a boat without a cox but because they did not appear to be proper amateurs.[57] Subsequent events were to confirm the alarms of the London men since it was the same Canadian crew that was to row Renforth's Tyne four for the professional championship of the world in 1870 and 1871. In 1876, London RC was one of three British crews invited to compete at the centennial regatta at Philadelphia. It proved to be a most unfortunate affair. The London RC four was fouled by its opponents and, obtaining neither sympathy nor redress, withdrew from the regatta amidst much recrimination. *The Times* wrote a sour report on the whole business, commenting that in America 'amateur was an elastic term and included coal-whippers, glass-blowers, hewers of wood and drawers of water'.[58]

It was London RC's growing concern at the conduct of events, both at home and abroad, that persuaded its committee to call a meeting of the leading clubs at Putney on 10 April 1878. Only the elite group were represented – Oxford and Cambridge universities, Thames RC, Leander and Kingston RC in addition to London. They did not meet to set up any kind of governing body, but simply to concentrate attention on what they saw as a single crucial issue, that of amateurism. Obviously, arriving at an acceptable definition would imply some kind of authority to enforce it but, for the moment, they avoided that conclusion. Given the membership of the meeting, the document that they produced was a predictable one, the logical consequence of the earlier attitudes of Selwyn, Shadwell and Egan. They also betrayed a debt to Brickwood since the first part of their definition was basically a paraphrase of his of 1866, suggesting that, at least among some, it had established itself as some form of convention. The 1878 rules began by asserting that an amateur must be: 'An officer of Her Majesty's Army, or Navy, or Civil Service, a member of the Liberal Professions, or of the Universities or Public Schools, or of any established boat or rowing club not containing mechanics or professionals'.

It concluded with a series of negative propositions to the effect that an amateur:

> Must not have competed in any competition for either a stake, or money, or entrance fee, or with or against a professional for any prize; nor ever taught, pursued, or assisted in the pursuit of athletic exercises of any kind as a means of livelihood, nor have ever been employed in or about boats, or in manual labour; nor be a mechanic, artisan or labourer.[59]

Here was a decisive break with the past. The lone views of the Dolphin Club sculler of 1839 and the powerful voices of his allies on the Isis and the Cam had become, apparently, accepted wisdom.

The timing of this initiative seemed totally justified three months later when four North American entries were received at Henley. Two of them appeared to be amateurs according to what became known as the Putney rules, exciting no comment apart from Columbia College's entry becoming the first overseas crew to win a Henley trophy. But one of the American scullers, G. W. Lee, was beaten in the final of the Diamonds by only the narrowest of margins and suspicions at the time about his pedigree were confirmed when he later became a professional.[60] Just as controversial was the Shoe-wae-cae-mette four from the United States of America who not only turned out to be lumberjacks but, according to *Bell's Life*, did not receive 'the plaudits bestowed on them with becoming modesty which is generally inseparable from true merit'.[61]

III

The cumulative repercussions of the Paris Regatta, that at Philadelphia and now the events at the 1878 Henley were to be of profound importance. The last, in particular, focused attention on the attitudes of the Henley stewards. Two issues were in effect rolled together, those of Henley's attitude to foreign crews and of their own view of amateurism. During a series of meetings between November 1878 and April 1879, the stewards considered the evidence, some of which revealed practices abroad opposed to the trends here in England.[62] For example, a letter from one of the French governing bodies, the *Cercle Nautique de France*, explained that all their amateur prizes were for cash, a form of behaviour that the likes of Brickwood would not have quarrelled with a decade or so earlier.[63] But the publication of the Putney rules, with their strong condemnation of any kind of monetary reward, had already closed that particular door and it is doubtful whether a single Henley steward would have defended such an approach. In the circumstances, the stewards decided that all foreign entries must be received early to allow some attempt at checking their credentials. Furthermore, they had to be 'accompanied by a declaration made before a Notary Public with regard to the profession of each member of the crew . . . and such declaration must be certified by the British Consul, or the Mayor, or the chief authority of the locality'.[64] Significantly, no mention is made of the foreign oarsmen not receiving any form of monetary prize but, assuming the secretary had the means of checking, he could advise the stewards to refuse an entry of which he was uncertain. But such a step first demanded that they themselves clarified their own position on the amateur question.

They had before them the Putney definition at their meeting of April 8 1879. It had not met with universal acceptance. As R. C. Lehmann recalled some years later, there was a significant gap between the positive and the negative propositions, one into which a number of oarsmen fell and who, as a result, were uncertain of their status.[65] The stewards, perhaps conscious of objections of this kind, decided to produce their own definition, phrased in such a way that everything was in the negative. It meant that it was made absolutely clear, as far as Henley was concerned, what kind of oarsman was not an amateur. The Henley rules, published prior to the 1879 regatta, declared that:

> No person shall be considered an amateur oarsman or sculler –
> 1. Who has ever competed in any open competition for a stake, money, or entrance fee.
> 2. Who has ever competed with or against a professional for any prize.
> 3. Who has ever taught, pursued, or assisted in the practice of athletic exercises of any kind as a means of gaining a livelihood.
> 4. Who has ever been employed in or about boats for money or wages.
> 5. Who is or has been, by trade or employment for wages, a mechanic, artisan or labourer.[66]

Unfortunately the exact arguments that led to the Henley rules must be a matter of surmise. The first oarsmen of any note to become members of the stewards had been H. H. Playford of London RC and Dr Warre, both joining the committee in 1868. Until the 1880s such men were in the minority and the stewards remained until then largely residents of the town and the immediate locality. At its meeting on 8 April, Dr Warre had given some indication of the hardline that he and some other former oarsmen were going to take in the not too distant future once they had obtained virtual control of the stewards committee. He announced that he would like the whole question of foreign entries to the regatta to be discussed.[67] In raising the issue, he was going straight to the heart of the matter. As he was to make clear in 1901, foreign competitors might not necessarily share the same values as those of the English oarsmen rowing at Henley. It, therefore, followed that to allow them entry might lead the stewards to look for a compromise on the amateur question. This is, in fact, precisely what happened. The arguments that persuaded the majority of the stewards to reject the approach of the Putney rules remain hidden. Possibly they recognised that to limit or ban overseas entries would seem churlish following Columbia's win the previous year. But much more important may have been the composition of the stewards committee. Still largely representative of a small Oxfordshire town and its neighbourhood, they may well have been flattered that crews from abroad wanted to row at their regatta. There was little indication of it happening elsewhere. Possibly, since they did not really appreciate the feelings of the leading English clubs, most of the stewards were prepared to take a generous view and to recognise that social conditions and values elsewhere were unlikely to mirror those in England. Their own definition of an amateur was, therefore, sufficiently accommodating to allow for entries from overseas crews. In making such a decision, they managed to produce a far more liberal document than might have been expected and, in doing so, they administered a salutary check to the pretensions of that relatively narrow group that had found its inspiration at the universities of forty years earlier.

IV

The consequent situation, however, could hardly be considered a very satisfactory one. There were now two separate definitions of an amateur, neither of them having the force of any kind of law, and both standing alongside the various different conventions adopted by the many regattas throughout the country. The situation of the Henley stewards in all this was paradoxical. They were now in the position of trying to enforce, internationally, rules that applied in this country for only three days of the year and then only over a limited stretch of the Thames. At no point did they suggest or encourage the idea that their own definition might have a useful application within the United Kingdom.

As far as the elite clubs and oarsmen were concerned, this particular Gordian knot needed to be cut. There is little doubt that many of them would have sympathised with an article in *The Times* in April 1880, that argued for the exclusion of working men and artisans from all amateur sports on the grounds that:

> the status of the rest seems better assured and more clear from any doubt which might attach to it and the prizes are more certain to fall into the right hands. Loud indeed would be the wail over a chased cup or a pair of silver sculls which a mechanic had been lucky enough to carry off. The whole pot hunting world would be so much the poorer to say nothing of the social degradation which the contest would have implied whatever its results would have been.'[68]

If this accurately represented the mood of many of the best oarsmen, then all that was required was a body prepared to enshrine such exclusive social sentiments into an authoritative code. Some noted that such a body already appeared to exist and, moreover, that it represented the particular clubs that had framed the 1878 Putney rules.

The Metropolitan Rowing Association had been set up following a meeting at Henley on 25 June 1879. Its headquarters inevitably were at London RC and it consisted of the same clubs that had drawn up the Putney rules with the addition of Dublin University. Its aim was a simple one: to form crews of the best available oarsmen to compete at Henley and to fend off any foreign challenge. As such it marked the formal conclusion of those indeterminate discussions of a decade or so earlier which had been part of Nottidge's legacy to London RC.[69] Although never called upon to form a composite crew, the MRA, embracing as it did the best and most competitive clubs in the country, seems to have attracted sufficient support to allow itself to be transformed in May 1882 into the Amateur Rowing Association. It retained the object of forming crews to meet foreign opponents but also adopted the larger aim of maintaining the standard of rowing throughout the country.[70] It was not surprising that its first headquarters were at London RC where for over twenty years the need for some form of controlling body had been under discussion. The original hopes of Nottidge and his associates had been sidetracked into the Metropolitan Regatta but, through London RC, had been revived by the establishment of the Metropolitan Rowing Association. But, once the new-found body had adopted what was claimed to be a national responsibility, then it had to find some way of resolving the central dilemma that there existed two definitions of an amateur.

As a purely voluntary body, the new association worked at first with some caution, so much so that *The Almanack* failed to notice its existence until 1885 and then only after it had reached a decision on the amateur issue. Its immediate preoccupation was with the visit during 1882 of the

Hillside four from the USA. Challenged by the Americans to produce a crew, the ARA declined, leaving it in the end to Thames RC to arrange a race. The American visitors were almost certainly without blemish as far as their status was concerned but their arrival had raised sensitive questions about amateurism and the proper mode of behaviour. They were perhaps a little unfortunate since they came in the aftermath of a controversial tour of Europe by a Cornell University four the previous year. The fact that the Cornell stroke may have deliberately lost a race in Vienna so as to gain financially from bets laid at home in Ithaca had left a bitter taste.[71] In its first public venture, the ARA was not to be tempted.

By 1883 the ARA was trying gently to extend its brief, announcing that it 'would proceed to exercise a thorough supervision over all matters connected with *bona fide* amateur rowing and be the means of settling any disputed points that may from time to time arise'.[72] But it was not until the next year that it turned its attention to the fundamental question of making a decision on the amateur issue. The ARA published its draft definition on 1 July 1884, following a meeting at Henley during regatta week. It is difficult to avoid the conclusion that there must have been some close consultation with the stewards, although nothing is officially recorded. That the ARA rules differed only marginally from those produced at Henley in 1879 underlined how crucial it was that the national definition should be basically the same as that being demanded of overseas crews. If the members of the ARA committee had decided to endorse a version of the 1878 rules, which, given the background of its members, it might instinctively have been expected to do, then its own credibility as well as that of the Henley stewards would have been seriously weakened. Instead, the draft made only small amendments to the Henley rules. They acknowledged that some amateurs might unwittingly have rowed with or against a professional for a money prize and it was agreed that they should not be penalised. Somewhat harshly and unnecessarily the phrase 'and anyone engaged in menial duty' was added to the manual labour clause. An additional sixth clause stated that nobody could be an amateur who 'was a member of a boat or rowing club containing anyone liable to disqualification under the above rules'. It was this last clause that was to prove the most contentious and controversial.[73]

The draft definition was circulated to interested clubs and regattas and, during May 1885, the ARA considered the replies. Those from the West Country and the Midlands revealed customs and usages that would apparently have meant the disqualification of a significant number of oarsmen. They asked for time to reconsider their position and this the ARA agreed by dropping the new clause for a year. It was never to be restored.[74] *The Field*, reflecting the views of some of the increasingly irritated elite group, took a tougher and far less generous line, claiming that, without the threat of the sixth clause, provincial behaviour, in particular, would remain unreformed and unpredictable. It had no doubt that the blame was to be borne, not by the small immature ARA, but by the stewards at Henley: 'to whose legislation exception can be justly taken more often than not'.[75]

In fact the ARA had behaved in making its first really crucial decision with considerable political sense. It had allied itself closely with the stewards at Henley and was in the process of cementing what was to become a powerful entente, recognised by the fact that, alone of regattas in this country, Henley has never been asked to affiliate. At the same time, the ARA had managed to avoid what threatened to be a provincial revolt that would almost certainly have destroyed the new association at the outset. It was clear that, if it was to survive with any degree of authority, it would have to behave in an expedient and tolerant manner. By 1888 twenty-four regattas had affiliated and agreed to enforce the ARA codes of practice, although others, while claiming to conform, had their own interpretations of the amateur rule. It was the West Country and Midland regattas that appeared the most contrary. Worcester had adopted the ARA code but its rules of racing did not completely conform in every detail. Evesham insisted on its own definition of an amateur, while Stratford-upon-Avon apparently ignored the issue altogether. On the upper Thames, Wargrave Regatta was not held under any recognised rules at all and allowed events for women as well as for men.[76] The ARA had been cautioned that it would take time for many to conform. In his comments on the draft definition, the secretary of Tewkesbury Regatta had bluntly warned that certain customs and practices would 'shock the delicate feelings of the lavender-gloved amateur; but if rowing is to be encouraged, we must not be too thin-skinned'.[77]

V

Irregularities and deception there certainly were from the strict point of view of the ARA's definition of an amateur. But a good many clubs and regattas would no doubt have seen them in a different light. The message from the Tewkesbury Regatta committee clearly reminded the ARA that custom and usage could not be abandoned immediately. The fear among some of the hardliners was that they would never be changed as long as the ARA persisted in what looked like its spirit of over-generous compromise. *The Field*, in particular, reflected the views of those who saw the behaviour of the ARA as unsatisfactory and it took pleasure in advertising faults and errors that came to its notice. In October 1888, it published a review of the rowing season 'showing the laxity which prevails, and the necessity for some stronger action in regard both to the clubs committing these breaches of the rules and the committees which permit them to be perpetrated'.[78] It was a theme taken up the next year in *The Almanack*, perhaps not surprisingly since it was published under the imprint of *The Field*. The editor commented that: 'there were some unsatisfactory doings in connection with the entry of "pseudo-amateurs" at the English regattas which were supposed to be confined to *bona fide* amateurs'.[79]

The faults were of two kinds. The first were those breaking the agreed rules of racing produced by the ARA in 1885.[80] Some of them appeared to be little more than technicalities such as the committee of Barnes and Mortlake Regatta allowing a man to row in incorrect clothing. But frequently, as in this particular case, *The Field* suspiciously detected far greater faults, pointing out that, during the previous year, the same man's entry for the Wingfield sculls had been refused. Such hints became serious accusations when it appeared that a number of regattas were allowing men to row who were not amateurs according to the ARA definition. Among those named was Bedford Regatta, affiliated to the ARA, as well as others that were not, including Evesham, Worcester, Southampton and Stratford-upon-Avon. The last caused particular concern. As well as rowing, there were bicycling and athletic events, the programme stating clearly that they held under the rules of the National Cycling Union and the Amateur Athletics Association. But, as far as the rowing was concerned, not only was there no mention of the ARA but the word amateur did not appear anywhere on the official card. At the same time, a number of other clubs were named for breaking the amateur rule. They were largely from the Midlands area but, *The Field* concluded, enquiries of Royal Chester RC, represented on the ARA committee, would no doubt have added to the list.[81]

Two weeks later, *The Field* returned to the issue, instancing the apparent problems experienced in athletics, swimming and cycling because of the slackness of their amateur definition. It reported with some relish two incidents where first a swimmer and then an athlete, both professionals, had entered for amateur events under assumed names. Both had been brought before the courts and sentenced to short terms of imprisonment. *The Field* had no doubt that 'these results are all attributable to the lowering of the status of the amateur, and it is in order to prevent rowing from falling to the same level, owing to the same cause, that the ARA is asked to devise a remedy. Should it be an effective one, it is not too much to hope that it may be adopted in other branches of sport.'[82] What *The Field* was doing was to reflect the sentiments of the most hidebound of the elite group who still saw the actions of the ARA in 1884–5 as producing the most unsatisfactory of compromises. They went further by claiming that anyone who did not fit exactly the terms of the ARA definition must be a professional, or, at best, a pseudo-amateur, someone in short who was claiming a fictitious status as an amateur.[83]

Such harsh and socially exclusive views did little to ease the ARA's burden or to improve its image among the many who remained suspicious and uncertain. Its alliance with the Henley stewards, a wise and sensible enough arrangement, could be seen by some as unholy, nothing more than a calculated piece of expediency, largely dictated by the foreign question. But the real danger was a different one that was to remain for some years to come. With its roots deep in the attitudes of the universities and the elite metropolitan clubs, the worry was that, under pressure from its more rigid and tenacious members, the ARA might revert to type and become simply the representative organisation of the praetorian guard.

VI

It was against this background, a beleaguered ARA and continued uncertainty about the real meaning of amateurism, that prompted a number of individuals to consider the setting up of an alternative body. Among them was Quintin Hogg, the merchant and philanthropist who, in 1882, had established in London a Youth's Christian Institute from which developed the Regent Street Polytechnic. Also closely involved were a number of Cambridge-educated clergymen whose rowing credentials were impeccable. Two of them, Sidney Swann and C. J. Bristowe had won blues at university and twice won the Grand as well as the Stewards at Henley, the latter subsequently becoming a well-known Boat Race coach. Another Anglican priest, P. S. G. Probert, a college oarsman at Cambridge, had also won the Grand on two occasions as a member of Thames RC. But towering above them in terms of personality was the formidable figure of Dr F. J. Furnivall. As an undergraduate at

Trinity Hall, he had rowed with some enthusiasm and built his own keelless sculling boat.[84] He became a scholar of wide and catholic tastes, a close friend in his youth of Charles Kingsley, Thomas Hughes and F. D. Maurice whose ideals he admired but set in a wide social context.[85] Furnivall was long connected with the London Working Men's College, founded by Maurice in 1854 and where Hughes taught and lectured for a number of years. A not altogether easy person, Furnivall was remembered by the young G. M. Trevelyan in 1903 as a man 'with a smile half benevolent, half Mephistophelean, permanently fixed on a red face framed in shaggy white hair; he was revered but not approved by the more responsible chiefs of the College'.[86] He never lost his love of the river and founded his own sculling club, encouraged women to row and delighted in the company of the less privileged whom he attracted to its premises at Hammersmith.[87]

The attempt to debar oarsmen by means of the manual labour clause was just the kind of issue to arouse all Furnivall's indignant enthusiasm. He aimed his attack at the universities, isolating what he saw as the misconceived twisting of those ideals that he had first met while a student at Cambridge and which had helped to shape his life. 'We feel,' he wrote:

> that for a University to send its earnest intellectual men into an East-end or other settlement to live with and help working-men in their studies and sports, while it sends its rowing men into the A.R.A. to say to these working-men, 'You're labourers; your work renders you unfit to associate and row with us', is a facing-both-ways, an inconsistency and contradiction which loyal sons of the University ought to avoid.[88]

It was sentiments of this nature that led on 5 September 1890 to a meeting at Ye Old Bell at Doctors Common that set up the National Amateur Rowing Association with its headquarters at the Regent Street Polytechnic.[89]

Its first act was to publish its own status definition in October 1890 to the effect that:

> an amateur is one –
> 1. Who has never competed for a money prize, declared wager, or staked bet.
> 2. Who has never taught, pursued or assisted in the practice of rowing or other athletic exercise as a means of pecuniary gain.
> 3. Who has never knowingly or without protest taken part in any competition with anyone who is not an amateur.
> 4. Who has never been employed in or about boats or boathouses as a means of pecuniary gain.
> 5. Who has never sold or realised on any prize won by him.[90]

What this statement made abundantly clear was that the new NARA was determined to have nothing at all to do with professional rowing in any shape or form and that its only quarrel with the ARA was its approach to the amateur issue. With that in mind, its first major decision in December 1890 was to appoint a small committee 'to meet representatives of the A.R.A. with respect to the definition of an amateur'.[91]

It perhaps gives some indication of the still uncertain authority of the ARA that it agreed to talk to what looked like a rival organisation. The meeting took place at Oxford in April 1891.[92] The NARA cause seems to have been unexpectedly deferential given the mood in which the new association had been founded. One of its delegates, F. J. Vincent, unable to be present, wrote a letter instead, the only existing indication of the way the NARA had decided to present its case. He did not, in fact, wish the ARA to abolish the manual labour clause since 'I am open-minded enough to understand and appreciate the object of some such classes being barred; the condition of athletics and football form arguments which only those who are wilfully blind cannot see.' All he asked for was some modification of the ARA rules so that they did

> not exclude men who are only disqualified by reason of their having rowed with or against the mechanics classes. The importance of this is so manifest in the provincial towns that I am convinced any member of the A.R.A. who knows the provinces will agree with us. We want to row with or against one another whether we are in trade or in a profession; whether we are clerks or engaged in mechanical work; and we do not want those who are eligible under the laws of the A.R.A. to be disqualified simply because they have taken part in a regatta or belong to a club in which there must always be somebody not eligible under the A.R.A. restrictions.

He concluded by saying that what the NARA would like was a two-tier system: 'I want the N.A.R.A. to represent the people and the A.R.A. the aristocracy. Let the men of the A.R.A. help in the larger association, but at the same time keep their own inner circle free, as it always has been, from any suspicion of taint.'[93] It was an unexpected case but, apparently, its arguments were undermined by the somewhat bullish and undiplomatic behaviour of Dr Furnivall, and the ARA firmly rejected the proposal.[94]

VII

The failure of the Oxford meeting prompted the NARA in July 1891 to issue a manifesto explaining its position. It specifically denied that it intended causing 'friction with any other Amateur Rowing Association' and stressed that it wished to work in harmony 'to maintain a high standard in the sport for the general welfare of amateur rowing'.[95] Its explanation seemed to reinforce its stance at the Oxford meeting. But the deference shown towards the ARA might at the same time suggest that clubs and oarsmen were showing some reluctance to join the new association, a view reinforced a year later by the Amateur Athletics Association's refusal to give the NARA any form of reciprocal recognition.[96]

Those who wanted some modification of the ARA's definition of an amateur found themselves in a quandary. W. A. S. Hewett, who had rowed in 1892 in the victorious Oxford crew and won the Grand at Henley, went to work at the Oxford House Mission in Bethnal Green, preparatory to taking holy orders. The plight of the oarsmen on the Lea, many of them connected with university and school missions, distressed him. They appeared to have been ignored by the Lea Amateur Rowing Association, established in 1881 and having close relations with the ARA.[97] In a letter to the ARA, he explained that there were clerks and such-like men who, although eligible to join the association, would not do so, preferring to row with their friends, many of whom were in manual jobs. Hewett was not impressed by the NARA and what he called 'the "heroics" of Dr Furnivall and the "brother-hood of man" sort of nonsense'. What he would have preferred was for the ARA to designate some regattas as first class under its existing rules and to allow the others to accept entries from any other kind of oarsmen other than professionals.[98]

A. B. Shaw, writing to the ARA from the Temple, was more sympathetic to the NARA, one of whose vice-presidents he was to become. He explained that he had considerable experience with many non-ARA oarsmen who 'row for the sake of rowing alone and are as much opposed to things objectionable in sport as anyone could wish'. Yet, confessing the weak appeal of the NARA, 'there are no other regattas at which they can or would compete'. He too wanted a two-tier system but this time of clubs rather than of regattas. He encouraged the ARA to recognise initially the clubs with which it had traditionally been connected but to allow others to admit any kind of amateur: 'If the A.R.A. could in each case see some guarantee against the intrusion of objectionable elements, it seems to me that they might admit mechanics to such clubs as these.'[99]

The Field, needless to say, took its usual robust view of the situation. Towards the end of 1893, it could write of the NARA as falling 'upon evil days, for we have not heard much of it lately, nor of its trumpery championships'.[100] This was an exaggeration. The NARA's real weakness was its virtual acknowledgement of the ARA's exclusive case and its hope for some kind of accommodation. If there was to be a change in the amateur definition, then it would have to be on the initiative of some of the ARA clubs and members themselves. There was certainly enough evidence to suggest that some of them would welcome some kind of modification. Two ARA affiliated clubs were angry and embarrassed that they were refused permission to entertain at their regatta the crews of Trent RC, most of whose members were working men but well known to the other clubs.[101] Marlow RC wanted the whole issue to be settled in as generous a manner as possible. Its captain, W. P. Wetherel, an Old Etonian, wrote to the ARA saying that:

> it would appear somewhat invidious at the present time, when all sports are so keenly taken up by the people, for anyone to say that one class contains more or better sportsmen than another. The spirit of the age – as I would that it were in all other matters also – is rather to weld all classes together by the community of their interests than to create or uphold invidious distinctions.[102]

The journal *Truth* took exactly the same view. It castigated the manual labour clause as 'one that disgraces any sporting rule. Briefly the case for the reformers is that the rule is arbitrary and unfair, and introduces unnecessary social distinction.'[103]

That the whole issue was becoming a matter of open debate prompted the ARA to appoint a sub-committee to reconsider the issue. Originally set up early in 1893, it was given a new impetus by the appointment of R. C. Lehmann as secretary in place of S. le Blanc Smith. Lehmann, a man of private means, had just missed his blue at Cambridge but became a coach of considerable ability and distinction. He was a writer of light verse, a member of the *Punch* round table as well as a radical in politics, standing for Parliament on a number of occasions before being elected at the Liberal landslide of 1906. In October Lehmann circulated the clubs and regattas about the sub-committee and asked for comments. It was in response to this request that Marlow RC sent the letter suggesting the abolition of the manual labour clause.[104] A number of others took the same stance, including Henley RC, Barry RC, Burton-on-Trent and, no doubt to Hewett's delight, the Irex Club from the Lea. But there was far from being unanimity and a number of the replies warn against assuming that the provincial clubs were of one mind. Some, like Leicester RC, complained of ambiguities in the rules and asked for clarification of the manual labour clause rather than its abolition. Others were suspicious about the possible consequences of any changes, echoing the view of Warwick RC, that 'considering the unsportsmanlike conditions to which other branches of athletics have degenerated where an extension of the amateur rule has been made, it does not appear that the time had yet arrived for any extension'.[105]

The arguments within the sub-committee are unknown but the cautious replies of some of the clubs must have reinforced the general conservatism of most of its members. Only two of the general committee voted for any change, while Lehmann added his own minority opinion in favour of some redefinition of an amateur. He made the point strongly that rowing was as much about skill as muscular power and he doubted whether the working man had in fact any built-in kind of advantage. He also applauded the opinions of Hewett and Shaw – without naming them but going so far as to use their actual words – and he concluded 'that the A.R.A. should take power to license clubs, without necessarily affiliating them, in order that they may compete at regattas held in accordance with the A.R.A rules'.[106] It seems clear that some kind of sensible and reasonable settlement of the issue was discussed and *Truth*, for example, saw some hope for the future in Lehmann's views.[107] But few had his vision and the main ARA committee veered away from such a liberal settlement. *The Field* reflected the majority opinion, commenting that 'it is a moral duty to be just before being generous. Justice to the amateur competitor in a muscular exercise demands that his opponents, like himself, should have developed their skill and anatomy alike by labouring for love and not for money.'[108]

Lehmann did not see this as a matter over which he should resign, remaining as secretary to the ARA until 1901. One explanation for this is that he had, in one crucial respect, had an important victory. Embedded in the full report, adopted as the ARA's policy in August 1894, was an exact definition of a professional. It was agreed that the word must be taken 'in the primary and literal sense', which meant that it applied only to those who actually made their living out of some form of rowing.[109] No longer would it be possible to brand an oarsman simply because he did not qualify under the ARA definition. But in fact the clause went further in its implications since it effectively conceded the demands made by the NARA delegates at the 1891 Oxford meeting. Basically, declared Lehmann, there were now three clearly defined kinds of oarsmen – amateurs according to the strict ARA definition, non-amateurs who were not professionals, and finally the professionals themselves.[110]

The NARA may not have been happy with the description of their oarsmen as non-amateurs but effectively its organisation and members had been given a form of recognition and those who qualified in either of the first two groups could now row together for pleasure or against each other in private matches, even though they could not compete in the same regatta events.

VIII

Lehmann's manoeuvrings had allowed the ARA to go as far as possible in accommodating the NARA. To have tried to enforce a complete relaxation of the amateur clause would probably have been politically impossible. It would have embarrassed the stewards at Henley whose goodwill and cooperation the ARA committee greatly prized. It would almost certainly have alienated the most vociferous members of the elite group whose skills the ARA were determined to encourage. But in any case there is little evidence that the NARA wanted to press its own case any further. Late in 1895, there was a suggestion that another approach might be made to the ARA but, significantly, it seems to have aroused little enthusiasm in the NARA executive.[111] The fact was that the NARA had implicitly been given what it wanted in 1894, a form of recognition by the ARA that left it free to continue on its own unpretentious way.

For the moment it looked as if the amateur issue was settled and the ARA could concentrate on the task of reinforcing its authority. By 1899, fifty-five clubs had become affiliated and, by 1913, the number had grown to eighty-nine.[112] The ARA was not much interested in the organisation of the regatta calendar and welcomed the appearance of regional associations and councils ready and willing to administer such arrangements. The Provincial Amateur Rowing Council, consisting largely of Midlands clubs, was in existence by the turn of the century and, until 1907, sent a representative to the ARA committee meetings. Council representation for the Thames was recognised in 1904 and the north-eastern clubs set up a similar body in 1911.[113] These subsidiary councils had the added merit of extending the ARA's influence to the non-affiliated clubs and ensuring that the amateur rules were more uniformly applied. The number that virtually ignored the existence of either of the associations was considerable. For example, from the ARA's list of 1913, only one club in the North East, Durham University, was a member. Those that remained outside presented something of a difficulty for which the ARA deftly provided an answer by suggesting that they might be treated in exactly the same way as foreign entries at Henley. Both York City RC and Leicester RC were told in 1906 that there was no objection to such crews being accepted at their regattas provided they applied by an earlier date than normal to allow their credentials to be properly examined.[114]

Slowly the ARA was beginning to increase its authority and exercise its influence. It made it clear in 1900 that regattas must not alter the rules of racing and status and that they were not open to local interpretation: 'even if the leave of other competing crews and of the regatta executive was previously obtained'.[115] The importance of such standardisation had been underlined by a dispute that year between the John O'Gaunt RC of Lancaster and the Mersey RC over inconsistent regatta rules.[116] The next year the principle was reaffirmed after Maidenhead Regatta announced that one of its events was open to, among others, the local volunteers, the yeomanry and the fire brigade.[117] Much of the ARA's time was taken up with considering the status of individual oarsmen. At one meeting in May 1895, for example, it concluded that, while an ironmonger, a paid tailor and an apprentice to a printer were not eligible, the booking clerk at the Great Western station at Henley was.[118] Nor was the ARA afraid to condemn a whole club because of its doubts about some of its members. In 1902, Evesham RC's request for affiliation was refused on those grounds.[119] This in itself did not prevent a club using the services of the ARA if it ever felt the need. It was in the interests of the ARA to show a degree of tolerant benevolence and to act as a kind of advisory agency. Durham ARC, a non-affiliated club, still looked to the ARA as the proper body to consult on a status dispute and on the possibility of having a women's section.[120] The reply is not recorded on the second point but it would certainly have been discouraging, the ARA having made its views clear on that issue in 1905.[121] Not that the evidence was always heeded. In 1914 Tees Amateur Boating Club, another that was not affiliated, raised with the ARA the question of whether being an apprentice compromised a man's amateur status. The Tees committee did not like the reply and accepted the application 'as he complies to our local rules the same as other members.' The secretary could not resist adding a note to the effect that 'it was reported that the following was the composition of a Nottingham crew which rowed at Henley this year – two painters, one butcher and a motor manager'.[122]

No doubt clubs did on occasions admit men whom neither of the associations would have approved of. But the fact that a non-affiliated club such as Tees ABC could seek the ARA's advice meant that it was conscious of the need not to step too far out of line. The time spent by the committees of both associations on considering individual cases suggests that, throughout the country, clubs were conscious of the need to be too nonconformist. Unfortunately few club minute books allow any close form of analysis of membership since they rarely state the

Table VI   *Durham ARC members 1861–94*

A. Professional, etc.		B. Tradesmen and Clerks, etc.	
Accountant	1	Baker	1
Agent to dean and chapter	1	Bank clerk	1
Architect	2	Builder	1
Assistant overseer	1	Clerk	1
Auctioneer	2	Clothier	1
Banker	2	Chemist	1
Barrister	1	Confectioner	2
Businessman	2	Fruiterer	1
Clergyman	5	General dealer	1
Commission agent	1	Miller	1
Dentist	1	Newsagent	1
Engineer	4	Tailor	1
Farmer	2	Tobacconist	1
Machine agent	1	*Total*	15
Medical	2		
Mining engineer inspector	5		
Private secretary to Lord Barnard	1	C. Manual Workers, etc.	
Schoolmaster	2		
Solicitor	15	Cartman	1
Stockbroker	1	Currier or mason	1
Tax surveyor	1	Grocer's assistant	1
Veterinary surgeon	2	Joiner or signalman	1
Viewer	2	Labourer	2
Profession not known but member of county or city council, J.P., commission in volunteers, university blue	4	Moulder or boat-hirer	1
		Prison warder	1
		Wood turner	1
Total	61	*Total*	11

Total: 86 out of 154 names in minutes (55.8%)
% of 86 =   A — 70.9%
          B. — 16.2%
          C. — 12.7%

Sources DARC *Minutes*; Durham School Register, Sunderland, 1968, 4th ed.; The *Durham Directory and The Almanack*, 1878, 1881, 1884, 1890, 1891, 1892, 1894.

Table VI cont. *Tyne ARC new members, May 1920 – May 1923*

A. Professional, etc.		B. Tradesmen and clerks, etc.	
Accountant	2	Apprentices –	
Architect	1	Draughtsman	3
Auctioneer	1	Drapery	2
Barrister	2	Engineering	1
Coal exporter	1	Cashier	1
Engineer	4	Clerks –	
Estate Agent	1	General	12
Medical	1	Bank	1
Merchant	1	Shipping	1
Quantity surveyor	1	Stockbroker's	1
Shipping agents & brokers	3	House furnisher	1
Solicitors	2	Ship's draughtsman	4
Teacher	1	*Total*	27
University students	4		
Welfare supervisor	1		
Total	26	C. Manual workers, etc.	
		Stevedore	1
		Total	1

Total: 54 out of 64 names in minutes (84.37%)
% of 54 = A. — 48.1%
　　　　　B. – 50.2%
　　　　　C. – 1.8%

Source Tyne ARC Minutes.

profession or job of those enrolled. Those of Durham ARC contain a list
of club members between 1862 and 1894 (Table VI) and the work of just
over half of them can be identified with some certainty. Throughout
those thirty-odd years, the membership seems to have reflected the kind
of place Durham was during the second half of the nineteenth century.
The large number of solicitors is not unexpected given the city's place as
the county town and the presence there of major law courts. Some 70 per
cent would have satisfactorily fitted the ARA's definition of an amateur,
while many in the second group would also have been acceptable.
Nevertheless, Durham ARC admitted a number of men who, on the face
of it, might have been debarred from the club by both the associations.
No doubt the distance from the Thames encouraged the club to have a

reasonably tolerant attitude, reinforced by the close-knit nature of a small cathedral city. It may well be one reason why the club remained aloof from both the ARA and the NARA until after 1945. The same was true of Tyne ARC but being unaffiliated did not prevent it from exercising a fairly strict control over its membership. During the early 1920s, its minute books named a man's job or profession and apart from one, a stevedore, those elected were eminently respectable in the ARA sense of the word. Most appear to have rowed actively for the Tyne club, unlike Durham where in a number of cases membership appears to have been largely a matter of local obligation. Such was C. D. Shafto, stroke of Cambridge in 1877, the year of the dead heat, who did not row a single stroke while a member of Durham ARC.

Given such circumstances, the ARA, in particular, moved with some care and rarely obtruded in local affairs unless some anomaly was brought to its notice. Before the Great War, it was equally careful and scrupulous on the few occasions when NARA matters came its way, honouring the conclusions reached in 1894. It had no hesitation, for example, in agreeing in 1902 that an oarsman who had previously rowed in an NARA regatta was still eligible to join an ARA club, assuming he had not infringed any of the rules.[123] The same point was reinforced in 1906 and 1910.[124] Meanwhile the ARA was sensibly making agreements with other bodies such as the Skiff Racing Association in 1902 and with some of the coastal clubs in 1913, once they had accepted the ARA view of amateurism.[125] Also during these years and parallel with the efforts of the Henley stewards, it was negotiating with various overseas bodies.[126] But these proved complex and difficult, presenting problems over which the ARA and the Henley stewards came near to tearing themselves apart.

Notes

1 Nottingham RC, *Minutes*, 27 October, 3 November, 8 December 1862.

2 R. W. Lee, *Oxford University and College Servants Rowing Club; Centenary Handbook 1850–1950* (typescript, Oxford City Libraries), pp. 1–2.

3 Anonymous, *The Record of the Rowing Club of St Philip and St. James, Oxford, 1889–1909* (Oxford, 1910), pp. 5–7.

4 *Durham County Advertiser*, 23 November 1860.

5 W. A. Locan, *The Agecroft Story* (Salford, 1960), p. 7.

6 *Ibid.*, pp. 7–8; C. S. Bell, *The First Hundred Years, 1879–1979* (Derby, 1979), p. 2.

7 Bell, *Hundred Years*, p. 4.

8 Lee, *Oxford University*, pp. 15–16.

9 Durham ARC, *Minutes*, June 1885 and *Letter Book*, 25, 26 June 1885.

10 A. A. Macfarlane-Grieve, *A History of Durham Rowing* (Newcastle, 1923), pp. 184–5.

11 Locan, *The Agecroft Story*, p. 17.

12 Durham ARC, *minutes*, 4 May 1882, 27 March, 22 May 1890, 2 July, 10 September 1891.

13 Macfarlane-Grieve, *A History of Durham Rowing*, p. 184.

14 H. R. Smith, *Dark Blue and White – The History of Evesham Rowing Club* (Evesham, 1948) pp. 6, 9.

15 Tyne ARC, *Minutes*, 10, 29 July, 1909.

16 Smith, *Dark Blue and White*, pp. 15–6.

17 Evesham RC, *Minutes;* 'Special general meeting', 20 August, 1908.

18 *Ibid.*, 11 April 1913.

19 *The Field*, 27 October 1860. R. B. Mansfield published a number of books during the early 1850s about boating trips on the continent using a gig. He combined them in *The Log of the Water Lily During Three Cruises* (London, 1873).

20 Charles Dickens, junior, *Dictionary of the Thames* (reprinted, Oxford, 1972), *passim*.

21 See for example, *The British Rowing Almanack*, 1873, pp. 113–26 with detailed guide to the Thames from Oxford to Putney. The advertisements at the end cover forty-nine pages, most catering for boat hiring.

22 N. Wigglesworth, *Rowing in the North West*, (unpublished M.Ed thesis, University of Manchester 1983), pp. 39–40, 68.

23 *Ibid.*, p. 71; London RC *Reports, 1856–68*, pp. 4–5.

24 Stratford-upon-Avon BC, *minutes*, 25 March 1896, 6 April 1903.

25 See, for example, Hollingworth Lake ARC, *Minutes*, 10 July 1873.

26 R. J. Davis, *Boating at Worcester in the Nineteenth Century* (Worcester, no date), pp. 10–11.

27 Exeter ARC, *Minutes*, 10 April 1901.

28 Tees ABC *Minutes*, 11 March 1922.

29 Stratford-upon-Avon BC, *AGM Minutes*, 8 March 1937; *Stratford-upon-Avon Herald*, 12 March 1937.

30 Evesham RC, *Audited Accounts* 1898; Durham ARC, *Letter Book*, 31 March 1890.

31 Durham ARC, *Letter Book*, 9 April 1902.

32 Durham Regatta *Minutes*, 20 May 1905.

33 Macfarlane-Grieve, *A History of Durham Rowing*, pp. 32–4.

34 W. H. Allnult, *Notes on the Oxford Regatta 1841–1891* Oxford, p. 7 and H. Cleaver, *A History of Rowing*, London, 1957, pp. 138–9.

35 Wigglesworth, *Rowing in the North West* (M.Ed. thesis), p. 22.

36 Argonaut (E. D. Brickwood), *The Art of Rowing and Training* (London, 1866), p. 151.

37 Locan, *The Agecroft Story*, p. 22.

38 Middlesbrough ABC, *Minutes*, 10, 30 April 1877.

39 Argonaut, *the Arts*, p. 152.

40 *Ibid.*, pp. 151–2.

41 R. D. Burnell, *Henley Regatta – A History* (London, 1957), p. 43.

42 Locan, *The Agecroft Story*, pp. 21–22.
43 *The Almanack*, 1862, p. 108.
44 London RC, *Reports* 1856–68, p. 2.
45 *Ibid.*, pp. 328–331.
46 *The Times*, 22 July, 1860.
47 *Bell's Life*, 29 September 1859.
48 London RC, *Letter Book*, 20 September 1859.
49 *Ibid.*, 9 May 1860. Casamajor's list of the principal clubs consisted of – OUBC, CUBC, London RC, West London, Kingston, Richmond, Ilex, Leander, Tyne ARC, Northern RC, Nemesis, Minerva, Royal Chester, Mersey, Clydesdale, Eton College, Westminster School, Radley College, Durham University, Henley RC, Cock Harbour and Cork.
50 London RC, *Reports* 1856–68, p. 148.
51 *The Sportsman*, 29 August 1865.
52 London RC, *Minutes* of meetings with metropolitan rowing clubs, February–August 1865. The clubs attending were London RC, Thames RC, West London, Ariel, Twickenham, North London, Corsair, Excelsior, Ilex, Nautilus, Phoenix and King's College School.
53 London RC, *Letter Book*, 15 July 1858.
54 *The Field*, 17 July 1886.
55 Metropolitan Regatta, Auditors's Reports – March 1872, February 1876, January 1879, February 1882; London RC, *Reports* 2 February 1885.
56 London RC, *From Strength to Strength – 1856–1981 – Portrait of London R.C.* (London, 1981), p. 10.
57 *Ibid.*
58 *The Times*, 13 September 1876.
59 R. C. Lehmann, *The Complete Oarsman* (London, 1908), pp. 248–9.
60 Burnell, *Henley Regatta*, p. 103.
61 *Bell's Life*, 13 July 1878.
62 Henley Royal Regatta, *Minutes*, 14 November 1878, 8, and 29 April 1879.
63 *Ibid.*, 29 April 1879.
64 *Ibid.*
66 Lehmann, *The Complete Oarsman*, p. 249.
66 *Ibid.*, pp. 249–250.
67 Henley Royal Regatta, *Minutes*, 8 April 1879; R. D. Burnell, *Henley Royal Regatta – A Celebration of 150 Years,* (London, 1989); pp. 4–6, 209–214 for the changing composition of the Henley stewards.
68 *The Times*, 26 April 1880.
69 *The Field*, 5 July 1879.
70 *Ibid.*, 20 May 1882; Lehmann, *The Complete Oarsman*, p. 151.
71 C. Dodd, *Henley Royal Regatta* (London, 1981), pp. 68, 91–2.
72 *The Field*, 30 June 1883.
73 Cleaver, *A History of Rowing*, p. 127.
74 *The Field*, 13 October 1888.
75 *Ibid.*, 10 May 1885.
76 *Ibid.*, 13 October 1888. Nor was Wargrave Regatta behaving any differently ten years later. Its regatta on 26 and 27 August 1898 contained just about everything except the normal kind of racing. Among some of the events

were – Tradesmen's Double Sculls, Watermen's and Tradesmen's Scratch Eights, Ladies' and Gentlemen's Double Sculls, Ladies' Double Sculls and a Tub-Race in which 'competitors must wear rowing costume or university bathing costume.' (Wargrave Regatta Card, 1898, *John Johnson Collection*, Bodleian Library, Box Sport 13).

77 *The Field*, 11 July 1885.
78 *Ibid.*, 13 October 1888.
79 *The Almanack*, 1889, 'Preface', p. 3.
80 *The Field*, 17 January 1885.
81 *Ibid.*, 13 October 1885. The clubs and regattas listed as breaking the ARA code and rules were – Huntingdon, Gordon RC at Gloucester, the Severn RC and the Avon RC, both of Tewkesbury, Bristol Ariel, Evesham, Worcester, Taff RC at Llandaff, Bute United from Cardiff, Bridgnorth, Stratford-upon-Avon, Bewdley, the Neptune and the Falcon clubs at Oxford, Warwick, Ironbridge, Leamington, Trent RC from Burton, Bedford, Pembroke RC from the Lee. In addition a number of coastal clubs were mentioned – Shanklin, Cowes, Ryde RC, Ryde Working Men's RC, Portsmouth Shovellors and Southampton Coal Porters.
82 *Ibid.*, 27 October 1888.
83 *Ibid.*, 13, 27 October 1888.
84 T. A. Cook, *Rowing at Henley* (London, 1919), p. 79.
85 Anonymous, *Frederick James Furnivall – A Volume of Personal Records* (London, 1911), p. 159; H. Bond, *A History of Trinity Hall Boat Club* (Cambridge, 1930), pp. 18–21.
86 G. M. Trevelyan, *An Autobiography and Other Essays* (London, 1949), p. 23.
87 Anonymous *Furnivall*, p. lxxx.
88 *Ibid.*, p. lxxix.
89 Cleaver, *A History of Rowing*, p. 136.
90 NARA, *Minutes*, October 1890.
91 *Ibid.*, 13 December 1890. The NARA members were Furnivall and messrs Robinson (Landsdowne RC), Middleton, (Nottingham Britannia), Vincent (Falcon RC, Oxford), and J. J. Lonnon (The Polytechnic). The ARA appointed J. H. Goldie (CUBC and Leander), S. le Blanc Smith (London RC and Leander), A. W. Nicholson (OUBC and Leander) and B. Horton (London RC).
92 *Ibid.*, 29 April 1891.
93 Cleaver, *A History of Rowing*, pp. 138–9.
94 Anonymous, Furnivall, p. 156.
95 NARA, *Minutes*, 9 July 1891.
96 *Ibid*, May 1892.
97 A. Crump, *A History of Amateur Rowing on the River Lee* (London, 1913), p. 13.
98 Cleaver, *A History of Rowing*, pp. 131–2.
99 *Ibid*, pp. 132–3. The exact dates of Hewett's and Shaw's letters remains uncertain but they appear to have been written in the months 1892–3.
100 *The Field*, 11 November 1893.
101 *Truth*, 21 December 1893.
102 *The Field*, 11 November 1893.
103 *Truth*, 9 December 1893.

104 A. Davis, *Records of the Marlow Rowing Club* (Marlow, 1921), p. 36.
105 Cleaver, *A History of Rowing*, pp. 130–1.
106 *The Field*, 5 May 1894.
107 *Truth*, 2 May 1894.
108 *The Field*, 5 May 1894.
109 *The Almanack*, 1895, p. 170.
110 Lehmann, *The Complete Oarsman*, pp. 254–5.
111 NARA, *Minutes*, 23 November 1895.
112 *The Almanack*, 1899, pp. 164–5; ARA, Published List 1913.
113 *The Almanack*, 1900, pp. 183–4; 1904, pp. 115, 193; 1912, p. 223.
114 *Ibid.*, 1907, p. 225.
115 *Ibid.*, 1901, pp. 180–1, 191–4.
116 *Ibid.*, pp. 187–9.
117 *Ibid.*, 1902, pp. 173–4.
118 *The Field*, 29 May 1895.
119 *The Almanack*, 1903, pp. 195–6.
120 Durham ARC, *Minutes*, 19 December 1913.
121 *The Almanack*, 1906, pp. 196–7.
122 Tees Amateur Boating Club, *Minutes*, 10 August 1914.
123 *The Almanack*, 1906, pp. 196–7.
124 *Ibid.*, 1907, p. 202; 1911, p. 210.
125 *Ibid.*, 1903, p. 197; 1914, p. 29.
126 *Ibid*, 1901, pp. 183–4; 1907, pp. 205–6; 1911, p. 207.

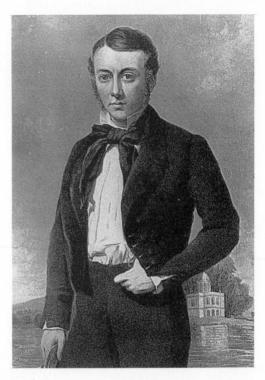

1 T. S. Egan

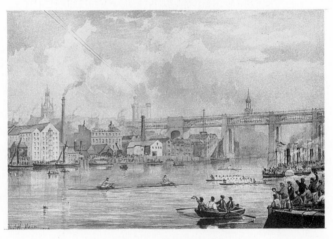

2 Sculling on the Tyne, 1866

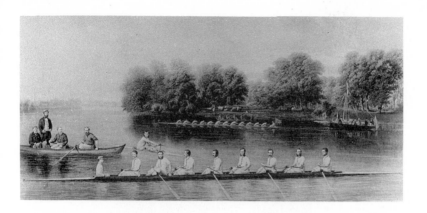

3 London RC oarsmen, 1860

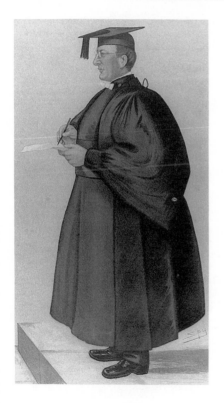

4 Dr Edmond Warre

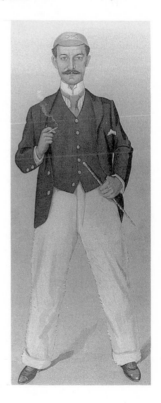

5 R. C. Lehmann

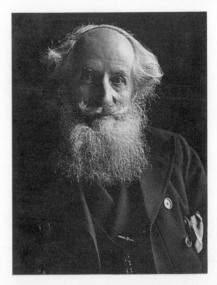

6 Dr F. J. Furnivall

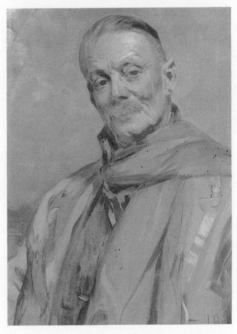

7 Steve Fairbairn

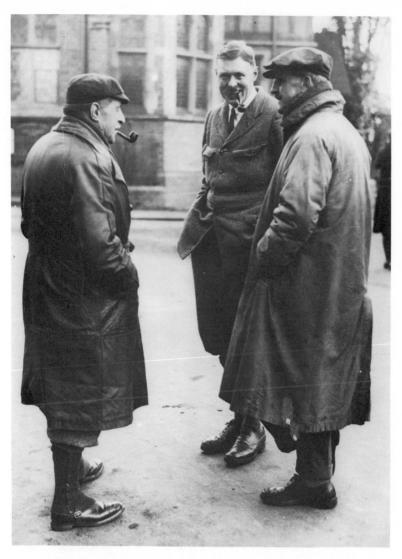

8 G. C. Bourne (with rowing cap), R. C. Bourne and E. W. Powell

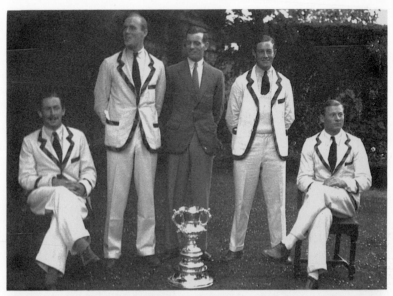

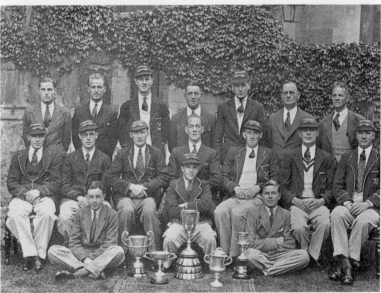

9 and 10 Contrasts – Jesus College, Cambridge 1932 and Oxford University and Colleges Servants RC 1934 – different associations but similar values

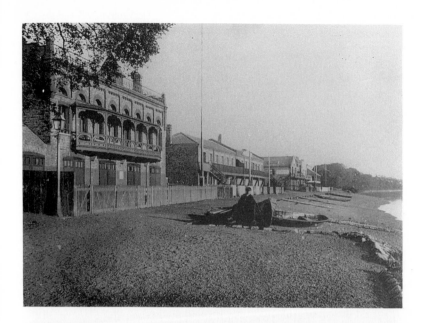

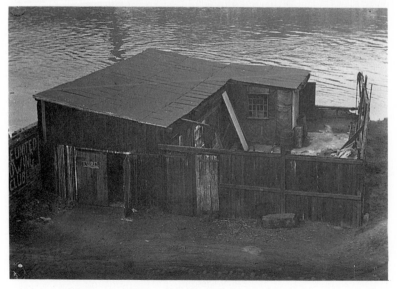

11 and 12 Contrasts – Elite Club boathouses at Putney Embankment and Tyne United RC boathouse at Gateshead

4

Little England – a slow demise

During the years before the Great War, while both the ARA and the NARA were trying to consolidate their authority, the issue of foreign crews visiting this country, particularly to row at Henley, began to loom larger. It was a sensitive matter that was of special concern to the elite group of clubs since on them would fall the responsibility of defending English rowing against such invaders.

At first they had welcomed the foreign challenge, especially London RC whose oarsmen went out of their way to organise matches on the Tideway against overseas visitors. During the early 1870s, these races rarely excited adverse comment. There was some question of the amateur status of the Atalanta four from New York in 1872 but that was authoritatively squashed by The *Daily Telegraph* when it announced that the Americans were 'what we in England are obliged to call upper middle-class men'.[1] These races were occasions that allowed a show of effortless superiority on the part of the English oarsmen, summed up by Frank Playford of London RC, following the defeat of a Frankfurt four in 1876, that 'no doubt they had seen and learned a great deal by their visit'.[2]

What had begun to sour the whole business and to sow seeds of doubt had been the very different experiences of English crews rowing abroad, particularly at the 1867 Paris Exhibition Regatta and at the 1876 centennial at Philadelphia. Such alarms had been subsequently reinforced by the appearance of some doubtful American oarsmen at the 1878 Henley. The major reason for London RC taking the initiative in formulating the 1878 Putney rules and stimulating the foundation of the Metropolitan Rowing Association the next year had been its alarm both about the amateur status and the rising standards of foreign crews. The Henley stewards had in their turn been forced by the presence of overseas entries to define very clearly their own terms of acceptance in a manner that seemed to contradict the narrow stance of the elite clubs. That the ARA, in 1884, seemed too readily to agree with the Henley authorities was a major reason why the most conservative of the oarsmen viewed the new governing body with some scepticism. It seemed to some that efforts to accommodate foreign crews and oarsmen were forcing both Henley and the ARA to compromise the amateur issue. When, therefore, some subsequent overseas entries at Henley did not appear to behave in an acceptable manner and seemed guilty of flouting the true amateur code, the temperature began to rise.

I

What was to become a crisis of major proportions was largely the concern of the Henley stewards. But it was in fact the ARA that prompted Henley to alter its rules. As part of its efforts to achieve greater credibility, the ARA was trying to establish mutual recognition between itself and foreign governing bodies. In 1892 it signed an agreement with the *Union des Sociétés Françaises des Sports Athlétiques*, a more narrowly-based body than its main rival, the *Cercle Nautique de France* that allowed amateurs to row for cash prizes.[3] A letter was sent to relevant regattas suggesting that entries from USFSA oarsmen should be treated exactly as if they were affiliated to the ARA. The Henley stewards considered this in May 1892 and agreed, that with effect from the 1893 Henley, their 1879 ruling would be modified to allow such French entries to be received on 1 June rather than on 31 March. It was accepted that in making such an arrangement, the stewards could not insist on the French entries being amateurs in the strict ARA sense but simply that they would be certified as amateurs under the rules of the French body.[4]

This double agreement with both the ARA and Henley was much appreciated by the French and through the good offices of their ambassador to London, W. H. Waddington, who was in fact a former Cambridge rowing blue, London RC was invited to send an eight to Paris in October to cement the new-found relationship.[5] Rowing in a damaged boat, they were promptly beaten, allowing the French rowing journal, *L'Aviron*, to crow with delight. Representative in the main of the views of the CNF, it suggested 'that our English friends must come down off their lofty pedestal'.[6] It was not quite the outcome that Waddington, his friend the Baron Pierre de Coubertin or the English authorities had wanted.

The incident, however, might easily have been forgotten had it not been for Thames RC, during a heat of the Stewards at the 1893 Henley, losing control of their steering and forcing their French opponents off course into a pleasure boat. The French immediately claimed a foul which Coubertin equally promptly insisted should be withdrawn. Nevertheless, the Henley stewards were greatly embarrassed, not least because they had been forced to summon a meeting just before the start of the regatta to consider a complaint by Thames RC about the amateur status of one of the French oarsmen. Only a personal letter from Coubertin had assured them that all was in fact well. Given these circumstances, it was a pity that Thames RC had not been able to steer a straight course. After an inquiry, the stewards exonerated the English crew from any suggestion of foul play. But there was an immediate outcry in the press on both sides of the Channel and what had at first looked like a promising initiative had degenerated into sad and unseemly charge and counter-charge.[7]

At the heart of this particular incident was the worry that, by being generous over the closing date, the stewards had not allowed themselves sufficient time to check the credentials of the French oarsmen. It reinforced the view that they were lax in enforcing their authority and that possibly they were not as rigorous as they should be in honouring their own rules. Such a view was compounded by the fact that, even with the earlier date of 1 March, there was not always sufficient time for a proper investigation. It seemed probable that a mistake had been made in 1892 when the Dutch sculler, J. J. K. Ooms, had won the Diamonds. The next year his entry was refused. The error was to be repeated in 1897 when the American, E. H. Ten Eyck, won the event. Once again, further investigation seemed to be called for and in 1898 his entry was turned down.[8] In behaving in this way, the stewards actually encouraged the kind of insinuations that might have been avoided had they been rather more careful in the first place. The secretary, in replying to Ten Eyck's club, the Wachusett BC, stated that 'my committee desire me to inform you that they considered the entry entirely apart from Mr. Ten Eyck's expertness as a sculler and presumed superiority over likely competitors at Henley, though they quite foresaw that such a reason for their decision might present itself in some minds'.[9]

Not all foreign entries excited adverse comment, even when they won, as Nereus of Holland did with the Thames Cup in 1895. But reservations began to be felt when crews from overseas were accepted for the Grand Challenge Cup, the premier event of the regatta. It was at that point that Henley began to be seen as an international affair and that raised for many in this country some fundamental questions about the nature of amateurism. Basically such foreign crews came with only one aim in mind, namely to win. In itself that was the main reason for the existence of the regatta but it was the single-mindedness of some foreign entries that was to give a shock to the system.

The first indication of this phenomenon came in 1895 when Cornell were accepted for the Grand. They were the best university crew in America and were coached by a professional, George Courtney. He insisted on the crew keeping themselves to themselves and made no attempt to hide the fact that he expected them to win. This sense of purpose was made clear in a heat against Leander. Through a misunderstanding, Leander were left standing on the stake-boat while the Americans went on to record an easy victory. To the delight of the crowd, Cornell were rowed to a standstill the next day by a little-fancied Trinity Hall eight. Cornell's fault was that, in their determination to win, they had breached the accepted code of conduct by not stopping after the mix-up at the start against Leander. They had not broken the rules of the regatta in any way but they were guilty of the kind of misjudgement that Henley found it hard to forgive. The point was underlined in the final of the Ladies Plate when St John's, Oxford stopped soon after the start when they saw that Eton had caught a crab. It was perhaps the only way that particular crew was going to be remembered – they lost by eight lengths![10]

Cornell's behaviour inevitably caused offence and called into question the advisability of continuing to accept such crews. One anonymous correspondent, recalling past incidents, wrote to *The Field*, asking:

> Did the performance of Lee, the Yankee sculler, tend to friendship? Did we gain anything from the dispute between the French four and the Thames R.C.? Do we love our American cousins any better because of the visit of the Cornell crew last year, with all the yellings and flag-waggings that accompanied it? I might add other instances, such as the Philadelphia Regatta of 1876 . . . When the international element comes in, sport ceases to be sport and is turned into a branch of foreign policy.[11]

By 1901 such sentiments were to be strongly echoed by others, more powerful and influential, as they saw the traditional approach of the main English crews in the Grand being seriously threatened.

The entry of Yale in 1896 caused no apparent problems. Nor did that of the Club Nautique de Gand from Belgium in 1900, though they pushed Leander very hard in the semi-final. The Belgians were to return the next year together with the University of Pennsylvania. Their opposition, apart from Leander, was not very strong, consisting of an average college eight from New College, Oxford, and two weak crews from London RC and Thames RC, both at that time going through a slump in their fortunes. There seems no doubt that had it not been for the presence of Leander, the Grand would have been taken abroad for the first time. As it was, they beat Belgium in the semi-final who then commended themselves by sending a bouquet to the Leander club house together with their best wishes for the final.[12] Leander, who had been together a mere fourteen days, then beat Pennsylvania, a crew that had been training together for over six months, by a length to keep the cup in this country.

II

No sooner was the 1901 Henley over when there appeared in *The Times* a letter from Dr Warre, a senior steward at Henley but written from his Eton College address. He made two main points. The first, which he did not develop but which was the major premise of his argument, was that he did not like international competitions since 'they take athletics from off their proper plane, and invest them with an importance which they do not deserve and ought not to have'. He then went on to claim that the donors of the Henley trophies had intended them for domestic racing and he hoped the stewards would reinforce that view, since 'I do earnestly desire that our amateur oarsmanship may be preserved from the deadly inroads of professionalism, which is already making a business of so much that ought only to be pleasure.' He concluded, without much conviction, by saying that, if foreign competitors had to be entertained, then no doubt it could be arranged elsewhere than Henley.[13] There was a voluminous correspondence in almost every newspaper following Warre's letter, including another in *The Times* from W. H. Grenfell, MP, a former Oxford blue, a notable athlete, and another Henley steward, stating that he had already given notice to the stewards of his intention 'to confine the entries at this regatta to the British islands'.[14]

Warre's letter uncovered a considerable degree of discontent at the way Henley had allowed foreign entries to be accepted. Sir John Edwards-Moss reported that he had declined election as a steward sometime earlier 'on the grounds that, if elected, it would be my first duty to propose a resolution to an effect similar to that of which Mr.

W. H. Grenfell has now given notice – practically a condemnation of the policy which those whom it was proposed that I should join had pursued'.[15] Others stated the case at greater length. W. B. Woodgate in *The Nineteenth Century* argued for allowing colonial crews at Henley even if the rest of the world was barred, which was just as well given the contribution at that time from a number of the colonies towards Britain's efforts in the South African War. He was happy to see an international regatta over the Boat Race course and thought that the Henley stewards might be persuaded to organise it. But his main point was that crews from this country were handicapped against the main foreign entries since the latter went for only one event, while the best English crews, including Leander, tended to double up in several.[16]

The most interesting and perhaps the most unexpected of Warre's supporters was R. C. Lehmann. Given his liberal stance in trying to find some accommodation with the views of the NARA in 1894, he might have been expected to show some sympathy towards the claims of overseas crews. He might, for example, have accepted the long-term implications of the hostile attitude of *The Field* five years earlier, when it argued that 'if the Henley authorities continue to admit foreign competitors who are not *bona fide* amateurs under A.R.A. rules, they cannot logically refuse admission to the same class of men from the British Isles, whom they now rigorously exclude'.[17] Important as this point was, it was not the one that the critics of Henley wanted to emphasise. For them the issue was less the amateur status of foreign oarsmen than their particular approach to competition, especially their clear determination to win at apparently all costs. 'The whole comfortable scheme of our oarsmanship would be disarranged', Lehmann argued, 'We should cease to look upon rowing as a sport: we should be forced to undertake it as a development of foreign politics. I can conceive nothing more detestable.'[18] He accepted that 'sport honourably pursued is, no doubt, a humanising influence'. But, he continued:

> when international rivalry comes into it, there is produced a tension of feeling, an excess, if I may say so, of enthusiasm which is apt to disturb all calculations based upon the placid character of ordinary competitions. Incidents which, if they occurred between two English competitors, might give rise to a passing flutter of emotion, are, in an international contest, distorted into a great quarrel; they give rise to angry recriminations and leave behind them a smart which years may not avail to soothe.[19]

It may well be that Lehmann, like others, had been brooding about these issues for some years, in his case, as he was near the centre of power, as secretary of the ARA. If Sir John Edwards-Moss is to be believed, the ARA had in 1899 warned the Henley stewards about foreign entries, presumably because of the difficulties of investigating thoroughly their amateur status. Lehmann was himself a steward and might have been expected to reinforce the ARA's cautious advice were it not for the fact that the ARA, in August 1899, appears to have changed its mind and agreed to continue negotiations with overseas bodies.[20] But Lehmann had one advantage not enjoyed by other members of the stewards in that he had some direct experience of how rowing was organised abroad. He had on three occasions during 1897–8 visited the United States at the invitation of the Harvard oarsmen whose rowing was at a low ebb, particularly compared with that of Yale. He had greatly enjoyed the experience, surprising the Harvard men by refusing to accept any kind of reward other than an honorary degree from the university and startling his friends by returning with an American wife. His success on the water had not been particularly outstanding, largely because he found it hard to graft the English notions of rowing onto the very different methods used by the American students.[21] But what he thought the visits had given him was some insight into the motives behind American rowing and he was not too impressed by what he had learned. In particular, Lehmann felt that he understood why the University of Pennsylvania had come to Henley and it was that crew's achievement in reaching the final of the Grand that was the immediate cause of the crisis. He argued that it was a problem of American university politics and that athletics were one way of gauging a university's status. If, Lehmann maintained, Pennyslvania had won the Grand Challenge Cup, they could not have been refused a contest with Harvard and Yale and the prestige of the whole university would have been enhanced. This, he continued, was the only explanation of Pennyslvania's single-minded attitude under their professional coach, Ellis Ward.[22]

As far as the Pennsylvania crew was concerned, the whole business was singularly unfortunate since all the oarsmen were still in the United Kingdom when the arguments began. They defended themselves as best they could, revealing at a dinner at Leander that they had been led to believe that efforts might be made to fix the draw to their disadvantage, something, they acknowledged, that had not happened. Lehmann was appalled, using the information to support his case, stating that Henley 'was not instituted in order that baseless suspicions of our fair play might first be created and then dispelled'.[23] A member of the

Pennyslvania faculty, J. William White, wrote to *The Times* in an effort to explain the approach of his own oarsmen, none of whom had rowed before going to university, and why a professional coach was necessary.[24] Nevertheless, the view persisted that Pennyslvania, like Cornell in 1895 and presumably also Yale in 1896, had been specifically trained with the Grand Challenge Cup in mind and that, although they were amateurs in the accepted sense, this constituted a professional approach which was alien to the traditions of this country. Only Leander, able to seek out the best available university oarsmen, past and present, could hope to match such opposition and, even then, they were virtually a scratch crew that by convention and inclination often rowed in more than one event. As it was, there were some among the metropolitan clubs who thought even that should be discouraged since it prevented former university men from rowing for London RC and Thames RC.[25]

Warre and his associates were not without their critics, who found an able and persuasive spokesman in T. A. Cook, a former Oxford blue, writing in *Fortnightly Review*. He took the approach that both Henley and the ARA had 'assisted in the education of the rowing world; and it would be a sorry ending if the mistress were to conclude her course of lessons by refusing to meet her pupils on the old terms.' He deeply regretted what he saw as an attempt to 'build a barrier round English rowing', an insularity that could only do harm. He concluded by asking: 'Does the whole scheme of British oarsmanship depend upon the perpetual presence in this country of certain ounces of inscribed silver?'[26] W. Dudley Ward, an old Cambridge blue, had already given an emphatic answer to such a question: 'If a foreign crew did win the Grand Challenge Cup, it would not be a national disaster. Let us be sportsmen with good sportsmanlike qualities, chief among which are fraternity, cordiality, and good fellowship.'[27] Uncomplicated sentiments of that kind represented the generous response of a significant number of oarsmen and clubs who were increasingly concerned at the possible turn of events.

The ARA had offered to discover, through the members of its committee, what the views of the major clubs were on the issue. These were reported to the stewards before its meeting in November 1901 when Grenfell's motion was to be considered. The vote was decisively in favour of foreign crews rowing at Henley. CUBC, Royal Chester, Kingston, London RC, Molesey, Thames RC and Twickenham all voted for the maintenance of the status quo, London's vote being by 280 to 92 and that of Thames by 125 to 38. Leander was slightly equivocal, stating that Henley was not a satisfactory course for international competition but that overseas crews should not be refused until contests could properly be arranged elsewhere. Only OUBC was in favour of Grenfell's motion but, again, the decision was hardly a decisive one. A tersely worded telegram had been sent to the ARA stating: 'Committee decided against foreign entries, provided they can row other than Henley.'[28] Given these circumstances it was not totally surprising that Grenfell was defeated at the stewards' meeting by 19 votes to 5.[29] A year later they considered a point made by a number of people during the debate and urged by CUBC in its reply to the ARA letter, that professional coaches should be banned from Henley. This was agreed, no such assistance being allowed within a month of the regatta except for scullers. An attempt to extend the ban to entries for the Diamonds was defeated the next spring.[30]

This was not, however, the end of the issue. The problems of foreign competition was to rumble on and, as far as Henley was concerned, there was to be yet another crisis in 1905, again over an American crew. This time the incident seemed to be more serious and not just concerned about motives or the nature of Henley Royal Regatta. The Vesper BC of Philadelphia was not a university crew but an ordinary club eight, one, by all accounts, of some speed and expertise. They were, as it happens, beaten in the semi-final of the Grand by Leander who went on to win the trophy. But, during the months following the 1905 regatta, it emerged that the American authorities had made scant enquiries before submitting the entry and that the members of the Vesper crew had accepted payment and been sent to England by public subscription. Such revelations were a serious embarrassment to the stewards and cast doubt on all their previous decisions over foreign entries, particularly their rejection of Grenfell's motion in 1901. The stewards were forced to face the problem head on and to take decisive action if they were to retain their credibility. They did so first, by forbidding Vesper to return to Henley, and then by insisting on new agreements with foreign governing bodies, ones that specifically demanded an acceptance of the Henley definition of an amateur. The immediate consequence was that only Belgium, Germany, Holland and Canada were in a position to sign, although other foreign crews could be considered as long as they could satisfy the exact amateur credentials.[31] For those who had for so long defended the ideal of the English gentleman amateur, it was a happy conclusion – the notion was now for export.

III

The 'Little England' view seemed to have been defeated. As far as Henly was concerned this was confirmed when a Belgian crew won the Grand Challenge Cup in 1906, repeating the success in 1907 and 1909. Indeed that trophy was to go abroad twice more before the Great War, Sydney RC of Australia taking it in 1912 and Harvard in 1914. To have tried to exclude such opponents after that would have seemed peevish and churlish. The issue was never raised again.

Nevertheless, in a different form, it was to continue to bedevil the authorities, particularly the ARA, for some years to come. International competition, as distinct from foreign crews rowing at a private regatta, was already well established. The *Fédération Internationale des Sociétés d'Aviron* had been set up in 1892 and the first European rowing championships were held the next year. FISA made a preliminary approach to the ARA about the possibility of affiliation in 1909 but the contents of the letter were simply noted.[32] A second invitation was received in the spring of 1913 at which point the ARA totally rejected such overtures, the reason being the obvious one that to join would have compromised the association's view on the amateur issue.[33] This was one form of competition that was to be ignored, a tradition not ended until after the Second World War.

The Olympic Games, on the other hand, were another matter, especially as those of 1908 were to be held in this country. The stewards at Henley were reluctant to entertain the rowing events over their stretch of the Thames and were persuaded only by their secretary who, keen to have them there, wrote an anonymous letter to *The Field* praising their virtue.[34] The main organisation fell on the ARA, not only to pick the crews to represent Great Britain but to ensure that the regatta was conducted according to the standards and rules expected in this country.[35] In fact it was a great success, British crews winning all the gold medals and all but one of the silver.[36]

Nevertheless, the terms and conditions of Olympic competition remained a source of continual worry to the ARA, conscious as it was of the kind of criticisms that had so lately been levelled at the Henley stewards because of their apparent generosity towards overseas entries. This fear, that it might compromise its own particular standards and be forced to waver on the amateur issue, was an abiding preoccupation. Its suspicions were not alleviated by reports that at both the London and the Stockholm Olympics, other sports had been guilty of breaking the

117

amateur rule, although *The Field*, never very generous when it came to praising foreigners, considered that there had been an improvement in many features of the games between 1908 and 1912.[37] But during the approaches to the 1912 Olympics, the ARA became aware of an apparent breach in the amateur code that seemed to have the blessing of the British Olympic Association. It was sufficiently concerned to issue a statement emphasising:

> that in view of the efforts that are being made in other branches of athletics to raise funds by public subscription for the expenses and training of competitors at the next Olympiad, this committee deprecates such actions as tending to professionalism in sport, and calls the attention of the affiliated members to the fact that under A.R.A. rules, oarsmen are no longer amateurs if their expenses are paid by funds raised outside their own rowing clubs.[38]

The question of how athletes should be funded and supported remained for the ARA the crucial issue as far as future Olympics were concerned. Although British crews had done well at Stockholm, retaining both the eights and the sculls, the ARA felt it necessary to repeat its warning of the previous year, since it 'viewed with apprehension the efforts which were being made in other branches of athletics to raise funds by public subscription'.[39] This was an alarmed reaction to a suggestion from the British Olympic Association for the setting up of a public fund to attract £100,000 for the next games at Berlin in 1916. It had some considerable support from, among others, Sir Arthur Conan Doyle and T. A. Cook, the only oarsman from this country on the International Olympic Committee.[40] Others, however, were more doubtful, including Guy Nickalls, a member of the 1908 Olympic eight, and R. C. Lehmann. They would have preferred to have had nothing to do with the Olympic movement at all.[41]

The ARA continued to be equivocal. Even before the Stockholm Games, its committee had expressed reservations about the future, informing the German Olympic authorities, in the spring of 1912, that 'they could not at this early date bind themselves to send crews to compete at the next or any future Olympiad'.[42] At least the ARA was consistent in championing its own particular cause. It refused an invitation late in 1912 to send a crew to compete in Australia, since 'they could not consider as amateurs those whose expenses were paid by any club or country other than their own'.[43] But, once the Great War was over, a representative squad was sent to the Belgian Olympic Games in 1920. It had first involved an unseemly argument with the British Olympic Association, which had also extended an invitation to the NARA to send crews.[44] Then, just before the Olympic Regatta for which it was entered, the ARA was asked to comment on a new constitution for the BOA. This gave it the opportunity of expressing, in no uncertain terms, precisely what it felt about the whole matter. Its letter stated: 'that organised international athletic competitions to take place at regular specific periods, and the expenditure of time and money which such competitions must necessarily entail, are entirely contrary to the true spirit of amateur sport'. It continued, saying 'that the exaggerated importance which is attributed to success in such contests endangers rather than stimulates the friendly relations which ought to exist between rival competitors and their respective fellow-countrymen'.[45]

IV

Such language might suggest that British participation in future Olympic regattas was unlikely. In practice, British crews rowed at all the inter-war Olympiads and with some success but, as far as the ARA was concerned, consent was given grudgingly. As the ARA told the Canadian Association of American Oarsmen in 1925, it 'had never been in sympathy with the Olympic Games or Olympic Regattas'.[46]

The root of the problem remained what it had been in 1901 over the question of overseas crews at Henley. What was at issue was a particular view of games and sports and the place they should have in society. Lehmann had no doubt what the answer was. 'Hitherto,' he had written, 'we have treated our rowing in the true amateur spirit, which regards the exercise not as the serious business of life but as an amusement for man's leisure.'[47] The fear was that international competition could easily mean that everything would get out of proportion. Hence the alarm about what its critics called the professional approach, with its emphasis on winning and on the need to devote excessive time to preparation, not least because such trends implied the provision of funds in some form or other to subsidise the atheletes involved. All this struck at the root of the amateur code where the slightest hint of monetary reward was regarded with profound distaste. It was the touchstone of the ARA's faith.

The NARA reacted in precisely the same manner when it came to questions of financial help or subsidy. But the similarity of approach on this particular issue did nothing to heal the breach between the two bodies. Just the opposite. In 1913, FISA had recognised the NARA as 'the only *bona fide* English association whose laws were compatible with theirs.'[48] Not surprisingly, in the circumstances, the British Olympic Association invited the NARA to nominate some competitors for the 1920 Olympics. The ARA was intensely irritated, commenting that the request had been made by 'a body known as the N.A.R.A. whose definition of an amateur is wider than that of the A.R.A. and consequently wider than that required of English competitors by the rules of the Olympic Regatta'.[49] The mode of reference to the NARA was ungracious in the extreme and the attempt to interpret Olympic rules in terms favourable only to the ARA was nonsense. But the relations between the two associations were already sour following the decision of the Henley stewards to refuse the entry of a NARA eight, made up of men who had fought in the war, for the main event at the Henley Peace Regatta in 1919. *The Times* referred to 'this pedantic regulation' and hoped that the rules governing amateurism might quickly be changed.[50] But such was the combination of circumstances that there was no likelihood of that at all. If anything, the relatively tolerant attitudes that followed the ARA's 1894 decision seemed to have disappeared. It was not, therefore, unexpected when the ARA decided in 1920 'that it is not advisable to alter the existing definition of an amateur'.[51]

The ARA gave every appearance of having absorbed, during the course of this long debate, many of the values of its most vociferous critics of the 1880s and 1890s. It gave the impression of becoming an increasingly obstinate and hidebound body. Yet the fact that someone like R. C. Lehmann, a man of liberal and often generous outlook, could be counted among its numbers warns against too harsh a judgement. The ARA and to some extent the stewards at Henley, were schooled in a particular tradition that was in fact originally inspired by Selwyn, Shadwell and Egan. Their standards remained those of an older generation. All the indications are that they would have preferred to retain the closed and intimate system that they had inherited and which had seemed at its best during the 1880s and 1890s. The incursion of overseas crews and the demands of international competition jarred, leaving many of them uncomfortable and ill at ease. Their suspicion of change was, in large part, a form of nostalgia and one which their own constituent members did not totally share.

The rank and file members of the elite group of clubs increasingly found themselves at odds with the views of their governing body. This lack of sympathy had first been seen in 1901 over the question of overseas crews at Henley. That attitude was to be extended when it came to participating in the Olympic Games and, in 1930 and 1938, in the

Empire Games. Such matters were largely the concern of the two universities and the stronger metropolitan clubs but occasionally also of a provincial club. In 1928, Nottingham and Union's coxed four was selected for the Olympic Regatta, only to discover on the eve of the first race that their cox was too light. At a subsequent meeting of the Provincial ARA Council, there was indignation at the failure of the ARA to pass on accurate information: 'Possibly it came through lack of interest in provincial rowing', was the sour comment.[52]

In fact such carelessness arose, in the main, from the ARA's lack of sympathy for anything connected with the Olympic Games. It was a form of discouragement that was to continue throughout the inter-war years and, even after 1945, had not totally disappeared. Sir Harcourt Gold, stroke of four Oxford crews during the late 1890s and chairman of both Henley and the ARA after 1945, shared the distaste of many of his contemporaries for the international aspects of rowing. But in G. O. Nickalls he had an aide of contrary views. The son of Guy Nickalls, who, in 1912, was unhappy about future participation in the Olympics, he had himself won two silver medals at the 1920 and 1928 games. He found himself frequently acting as deputy to Gold at international meetings since early on he had perceived that 'it did not take any particular foresight on my part to realise that the ambition of the majority of young men . . . was to succeed internationally and to set their sights beyond the somewhat restricted competition to be found in this country.'[53] To Warre, Grenfell and many others of that generation, such sentiments would have seemed incomprehensible.

Overseas rowing and international competition had had a significant effect on the amateur issue. The reaction of both the Henley stewards and then of the ARA – several of them being one and the same persons – during the late 1870s and the early 1880s had been to try to accommodate the problem where possible. In doing so, they had modified the notion of an amateur to the point where a much larger group, than might originally have been expected, were able to meet the ARA criteria, to the disadvantage in many respects of the NARA. But, assailed on the one side by those who would have preferred a more severe approach and on the other by doubts as they witnessed foreign values and practices that differed so much from their own, the officials at the ARA seemed by the 1920s to be back-pedalling. It had some unfortunate and unedifying consequences. The NARA was treated with undisguised contempt, while some among the praetorian guard made it clear that they did not totally approve of the ARA's rigidity. Cocooned in their own happy memories of the 1890s, the senior members of the ARA found themselves forced to accept the reality of international competition even when they largely disapproved of it. That its representatives undoubtedly rowed against some who were not amateurs in the strict ARA sense did little to commend their stance as far as domestic affairs were concerned.

Notes

1 London RC, *From Strength to Strength – 1856–1981 – Portrait of London R.C.* (London, 1981), p. 10.
2 *Ibid.*, p. 11
3 Henley Royal Regatta, *Minutes*, 25 April 1879.
4 *Ibid.*, 27 May 1892; R. D. Burnell, *Henley Regatta – A History* (London, 1957), p. 246. This 1892 change became the basis for future agreements between Henley and other foreign bodies.
5 Waddington was educated at Rugby and Trinity College, Cambridge, gaining his blue in 1849. He was, for a time, the prime minister of France, being one of only two rowing blues ever to have held such an office in his particular country, the other being Lord Bruce of Melbourne (CUBC 1904).
6 Quoted in *The Field*, 8 October 1892.
7 Henley Royal Regatta, *Minutes*, 27 May 1892, 24 June, 1 July, 7 July 1893.
8 *The Field*, 8 October 1892; T. A. Cook, *Fortnightly Review*, October 1901, p. 650.
9 Henley Royal Regatta, *Minutes*, 16 May, 1898.
10 Burnell, *Henley Regatta*, pp. 116–18; T. A. Cook, *The Sunlit Hours – A Record of Sport and Life* (London, 1925), p. 184.
11 *The Field*, 14 March 1896.
12 Cook, *Fortnightly Review*, p. 652.
13 *The Times*, 9 July 1901.
14 *Ibid.*, 15 July 1901.
15 *Ibid.*, 30 July 1901.
16 W. B. Woodgate, 'International boat-racing', *Nineteenth Century and After*, September 1901, pp. 439–48.
17 *The Field*, 2 May 1896.
18 R.C. Lehmann, 'Henley – and after', *New Liberal Review*, August 1901, p. 22.
19 *Ibid.*, p. 21.
20 *The Times*, 15 July 1901.
21 John Lehmann. *R.C. Lehmann in America* (unpublished typescript); T.C. Mendenhall, 'Coaches and coaching: the British are coming (R. C. Lehmann)'. *The Oarsman*, January/February 1979.
22 Lehmann, *New Liberal Review*, p. 23.
23 *Ibid.*, p. 24.
24 *The Times*, 25 July 1901.
25 *The Field*, 13 July 1901; 'The Leander fetish', *Truth*, 5, 19 December 1901.
26 Cook, *Fortnightly Review, passim.*
27 *The Times*, 5 August 1901.

28 *The British Rowing Almanack*, 1902, pp. 201–2; *The Field*, 30 November 1901.
29 *The Field*, 30 November 1901.
30 Burnell, *Henley Regatta*, p. 123.
31 Henley Royal Regatta, *Minutes*, 7, 23 June, 25 July, 7 November, 1906.
32 *The Almanack*, 1910, p. 208.
33 *Ibid.*, 1914, p. 237.
34 Burnell, *Henley Regatta*, pp. 131–2.
35 *The Almanack*, 1907, pp. 219, 220–24, 232–3.
36 Burnell, *Henley Regatta*, pp. 135–6.
37 *The Field*, 17 August 1912.
38 *The Almanack*, 1912, p. 226.
39 *The Times*, 21 December 1912.
40 *Ibid*, 27 August 1913, 1 December 1913.
41 *Ibid.*, 13 December 1913; *Granta*, 15, 22 November 1913; *The Field*, 17 August 1913.
42 *The Almanack*, 1913, p. 257.
43 *Ibid.*, p. 261.
44 *Ibid.*, 1920, p. 179.
45 *Ibid.*, 1921, pp. 146–7.
46 *Ibid.*, 1925, pp. 191–2.
47 Lehmann, *New Liberal Review*, p. 22.
48 NARA *Minutes*, 21 October 1913.
49 *The Almanack*, 1921, p. 179.
50 *The Times*, 1 July 1919.
51 *The Almanack*, 1922, p. 147.
52 *Ibid.*, 1929, pp. 173–4.
53 G. O. Nickalls, *A Rainbow in the Sky* (London, 1974), p. 170.

5

The dominant influence

The continuing debate about international competition revealed some considerable degree of tension among the members of the praetorian guard. Superficially all seemed well and the 1908 Olympic Regatta, in spite of all the misgivings, had been highly successful, while four years later at Stockholm, British crews had done well enough. But the ARA committee would have been appalled if victories at international level had been taken as the main criterion by which rowing in this country was to be judged and the Henley stewards would have agreed with them. There was, in any case, a degree of blustering about some of those Olympic wins that suggested all was not quite as it should be. The engagingly direct comments of Guy Nickalls, at forty-one the oldest member of the 1908 winning eight, emphasised his remarkable grit and determination, but at the same time placed him firmly in the Little England camp. Writing of the 1908 Olympic Regatta, he bluntly stated that he had never in his life been beaten by a colonial or a foreigner and that he had no intention of being so in his last race.[1] He had only consented to come out of retirement, along with a number of other relatively old oarsmen, because the alternatives open to the selectors had seemed so poor. The other British eight entered for the 1908 Olympics had been the Cambridge crew that had won the Boat Race a few months earlier. Nickalls could not hide his contempt at the manner and method of their victory: 'They could not very well have helped it,' he wrote, 'as at the time Oxford was even more devoid of oarsmen of merit than was Cambridge'.[2]

The decade or so before the Great War was a period of substantial tension both at home and abroad. On the surface, British society appeared prosperous enough, though the benefits were unevenly spread, but underneath there was considerable and often bitter unrest.

The same was true of the international scene. In miniature, the world of the elite group of oarsmen seemed in some ways to mirror these strains. The debate about foreign crews at Henley and the problems posed by rowing abroad had been informed by a particular combination of nostalgia and fear. Among many there was a tendency to look back over their shoulders to the 1880s and the 1890s and to compare the oarsmen and crews of the immediate pre-1914 period unfavourably with those who had gone before them. Warre, Grenfell, Lehmann and their associates may sincerely have believed that the values and ideals that had for so long governed their approach to rowing were in danger of being compromised, particularly their cherished concept of the amateur, but at the same time they managed to convince themselves that the younger generation of oarsmen were no longer as good as those of the immediate past. That they might be beaten by overseas crews was an unspoken fear, one that was realised in 1906 when the Belgians became the first foreign eight to win the Grand Challenge Cup at Henley. Yet it was this younger group of oarsmen who, in spite of their supposed imperfections, were more than eager to test themselves against any opposition, whatever its place of origin. Parallel to this debate was another, that over the methods and approach of Steve Fairbairn, the first arguments of which were to be heard before 1914, although it was not until after the war that it came to divide men into often hostile camps. It was all somewhat confusing as the elite clubs and their representatives seemed increasingly to be so much at odds with each other.

I

All these arguments were confined to the performances of those clubs that were at the heart of the praetorian guard. They remained as they had been since the last two decades of the nineteenth century – the boat clubs of the two universities and their constituent colleges, Leander, London RC and Thames RC with the likes of Kingston RC, Molesey BC and Royal Chester as the best of the second division. There is no evidence to suggest that they changed their membership in any dramatic way. They were basically middle class, normally from the public schools and often university educated men who had obtained entrance as much by the ability of their parents to pay as on their academic merit. David Haig-Thomas, bow of the victorious Cambridge Boat Race crews of 1930, 1931 and 1932 and a member of the Leander eight that won the Grand at Henley in 1932 and then represented Great Britain at the Los Angeles

Olympics, saw no particularly good reason why he should complete his three years at university by gaining a degree since neither his grandfather nor his father had bothered to do so.[3] Not that all oarsmen at the universities took quite such a cavalier approach to their academic responsibilities. Even before 1914, when the number of men taking an honours degree tended to be smaller than during the inter-war years, a good many of the oarsmen at Trinity Hall, Cambridge, managed in the sixty or so years prior to the Great War to do reasonably well in the Tripos, some outstandingly so.[4] Leander's membership continued to be exclusive, the great majority being university men, although, unlike London RC and Thames RC, the club rarely boated crews except for Henley Royal Regatta. The two main metropolitan clubs could, had they so wished, have taken advantage of the relatively liberal rulings of the ARA that allowed men of often humble background to join one of their clubs as long as they were not working in the boat business or engaged in menial jobs. There is, however, no evidence that they did so. There are no requests for clarification of a man's eligibility to row from either of the clubs in the available records of the ARA and, in any case, had such a man asked for membership, the social ethos of both might subsequently have inhibited him. But, unlike Leander, neither London RC nor Thames RC came to rely on a steady supply of university oarsmen, although they were only too pleased to welcome them when they came. In both of them the majority of members, like Thames RC's most distinguished inter-war oarsman, Jack Beresford, had not been to either of the universities, contenting themselves with posts in the City of London.

Attempting to judge the real worth of many of these clubs and their crews remains difficult. They still dominated Henley Royal Regatta. Of the fifty-five finals for the Grand Challenge Cup between 1880 and 1939, Leander won twenty-one times, the Oxford and Cambridge colleges thirteen, the two main metropolitan clubs on a further thirteen occasions and overseas crews had eight victories. In the Stewards, the senior event for fours, the university colleges dominated the event with twenty-four wins during the period to the eight by Leander. Four overseas crews were successful as were seventeen from the metropolitan Thames, including a single win by Kingston RC in 1884. Two non-metropolitan clubs, Royal Chester and Eton Vikings, the latter a club reserved for Old Etonians, also had victories. Whatever doubts there may have been about the foreign challenge, the elite clubs had done well in their defence of the two main Henley titles prior to 1939, limiting the overseas victories to just less than 11 per cent. In doing so, the part played by the two universities, in the inter-war period Cambridge particularly, was remarkable, especially when it is remembered that many of the Leander crews were constructed from current university oarsmen.

The arguments about how good these crews actually were was, nevertheless, a fierce one. In large measure it came down to a discussion of style and what was the best means of propelling a boat quickly through the water. G. C. Bourne, himself a former Oxford blue and coach of many Oxford crews from the mid-1880s until the late 1920s, had no doubt that the 1890s marked the Augustan age of English rowing:[5] it was then that standards had been set and the orthodox approach had been seen at its best. Bourne also advanced the view that there was some kind of inevitability about variations in standards, just as trade booms and depressions appeared to follow one another with a certain monotonous regularity. He had no doubt that the reason for this was that certain facets of the rowing stroke began to be over-emphasised, so that 'though the evil effects of exaggeration are soon manifest, the enthusiasts continue to apply their favourite nostrum with so little discretion that the final result is incompetence'.[6] There is no doubt that he was correct in this analysis though he was perhaps a little unkind in his criticisms of those who tried to find a remedy, so much so that he refused to name the university responsible for supporting heretical practices. He claimed that at one of them 'the theory of discarding all superfluity of adornment in rowing and concentrating on essentials was for a while conspicuously successful. Presently the desire to avoid exaggeration became itself an exaggeration . . . Drastic remedies and a long and severe course of discipline were required to stop the rot.'[7] Given the criticisms made at the time, Bourne's strictures might have applied equally to either of the universities since both for a period before 1914 departed from orthodox norms. The three winning Cambridge crews between 1906 and 1908, stroked by D. C. R. Stuart, met with little real approval from anybody except R. C. Lehmann, the last of them being the Olympic eight so mocked by Guy Nickalls.[8] They appear to have used what some contemporaries described as a sculling style, with the main emphasis being placed on a thrust of the legs in the middle of the stroke. Equally condemned was the Christ Church eight that in 1908 won the Grand at Henley. Coached by W. A. L. Fletcher, a member of several of those 1890 crews so praised by Bourne, its method of rowing appeared to be an attempt to copy those used by the Belgian crews. The official historians at the time of the centenary of the Boat Race, only one of whom could have witnessed either of these departures from the orthodox, were still incensed by what had happened as late as 1929. Their final condemnation of what had taken place at Cambridge could just as well have been applied to the Christ Church approach. Admitting that Stuart and his coaches brought their particular style to as high a degree of expertise as was possible, they nevertheless concluded, that 'to aim at perfection in only one of the cardinal points of oarsmanship, instead of in all of them, is treading the easier path'.[9] T. S. Egan would have rejoiced at such sentiments.

An anonymous and ironic comment on the whole situation in *The Spectator*, just before the 1907 Henley, declared that 'the principles of British rowing have almost become part of the constitution' and, noting that orthodox crews tended to swing the bodies in a manner avoided by the Belgians, concluded nevertheless that things ought to stay as they were if only to avoid the rewriting of the Eton boating song.[10] But for those most closely involved, the points that concerned them were hardly matters for levity and wit. For behind all these arguments and experiments was an important and fundamental issue, since the orthodox style had almost begun to assume the hallmark not just of a particular way of rowing a boat but of holy writ. Heretical views and methods were therefore treated with considerable suspicion, if not with open hostility. Factional divisions emerged whose supporters viewed each other with the intensity of religious parties, like Evangelical and Tractarian clergymen arguing at a diocesan synod. Particularly was this the case over the approach of Steve Fairbairn. An Australian, he had rowed for Cambridge in 1882, 1883, 1886 and 1887. There is a certain paradox, given his subsequent views on the inherent faults of orthodoxy, that in his first two Boat Races he was to be beaten by two of its greatest apostles, G. C. Bourne and R. S. de Havilland. From just after the turn of the century, Fairbairn spent most of his time in this country and devoted himself to the interests of the boat club at Jesus College, Cambridge. During the 1920s he also coached Thames RC and subsequently London RC, both with considerable success.

Bourne, whose *A Textbook of Oarsmanship* was published in 1925, became the leading protagonist of the older orthodox approach and he remains the most persuasive and elegant exponent of its virtues. But in drawing attention to the danger of exaggerating one particular element in the stroke, he was himself warning against some of the difficulties inherent in the gospel that he was preaching. R. S. de Havilland, in his reluctant criticisms of Warre, was doing the same. What seemed to be at issue was the emphasis on a man's swinging his body at the beginning of the stroke to the point where he could confuse length of stroke with what was really, as one critic called it, 'exhausting overreach'.[11] The argument was that such a manner of rowing was inefficient, since a man might use so much energy in releasing himself from this position that he could not effectively use his legs, the most powerful muscles in an oarsman's body. The much maligned D. C. R. Stuart commented that many orthodox coaches 'will have it that swing must be taught first, foremost, and at all times, and leg work left to take care of itself'.[12] There seems little doubt that this was true of some crews of that school whose oarsmen and coaches managed to produce parodies of a highly success-ful method. It is significant that in writing his book, Bourne makes no reference to the controversies aroused by Fairbairn but simply pays due reverence to the teaching of Warre, claiming that 'my attempt to push the analysis of the stroke to the farthest limits of which I am capable has resulted in a complete vindication of the principles which he laid down for the guidance of all future generations of oarsmen'.[13] By implication, he was admitting that the orthodox method could be abused and that in the hands of the less sensitive could become stale, fossilised and not all that profitable. As one waggish versifier put it, a trifle unfairly as far as Bourne was concerned:

> Beware the Orthodox, my son,
> The slides that check, the arms that snatch;
> Beware the drop-in blade, and shun
> The Bourneish shoulder-catch.[14]

Fairbairn would, no doubt, have equally wished to disown some of the crews that appeared under his particular banner, the consequence of not very intelligent coaches who used his words without really understand-ing what he was trying to do. After watching the splendid final of the Grand Challenge Cup in 1932 when the Cambridge eight rowing as Leander beat Thames RC by a third of a length, the one supposedly a fine example of an orthodox crew and the other of the Fairbairn school, S. M. Bruce wrote to *The Times* saying that he had been unable to distinguish between them as far as style was concerned: 'The whole trouble arises from the unsound teaching of many who claim to be the advocates of either one or the other.'[15] Fairbairn must have been delighted with such a comment, leaving aside the fact that it came from another Australian, since he always claimed he was not interested in style but in method. He once wrote that 'styles in rowing are like seasons in Australia, bad, damned bad and bloody awful'. What he was anxious to encourage was a positive and intelligent approach in which a man would try to think out for himself the best way of moving a boat.[16] It should not have surprised him that Bourne would have been in entire agreement. He wrote in the preface to his book that 'it is, to my way of thinking, intolerable that a Wrangler should row in a University boat and not bother himself to inquire into the principles on which his oarsmanship depends'.[17]

II

These arguments and misunderstandings were to go on for several more years, well after Fairbairn died in 1938. In 1952 R. D. Burnell could publish his *Swing Together* which still saw English rowing in terms of a clash between the protagonists of the two sides, although he was careful to distinguish between what he saw as true Fairbairnism and the style practised by Jesus College crews at that time, what he called 'an appalling caricature of rowing'.[18] Six years later, Peter Haig-Thomas, coach of most of the inter-war Cambridge crews, could write *The English Style of Rowing* together with M. A. Nicholson who looked after the eight at Eton. It was a robust and intelligent defence of orthodoxy that attacked not just the same terrible manifestations that had so upset Burnell when he looked at the Jesus crews but also criticised the equally odd developments encouraged by Roy Meldrum as coach of the Lady Margaret crews at Cambridge.[19] Yet, when they were published, these two books proved in fact to be the funeral orations on both sides as different and far more radical methods were being developed elsewhere on the continent that were totally to alter the approach of coaches and oarsmen. Nevertheless, the fact that rowing in this country could during the 1950s still be discussed in terms that pre-dated the Great War emphasises the very real depth of feeling that was felt on these issues. The symbol for many of true orthodoxy was the fixed rowing-pin, as powerful a badge as ever the true cross had been to the medieval crusaders. In 1935 the Cambridge president, M. Bradley, decided to use swivel rowlocks, the kind used by all Fairbairn crews, and so upset were two of CUBC's longstanding coaches, Peter Haig-Thomas and F. J. Escombe, that, like T. S. Egan of old, they immediately offered their services to Oxford.[20] With hindsight the arguments now seem irrelevant and even trivial, yet men with great loyalty to their university and its boat club were prepared to abandon that allegiance on a point of principle. It deserves some form of explanation.

From one point of view it looks a little like simple obstinacy, the old guard being determined to resist the new ideas of the young Turks whose views made them feel uncomfortable and uneasy. Like the arguments over foreign crews at Henley and the international aspect of rowing, the resistance was a compound of regret at the apparent passing of a golden age and fear that, without a return to old virtues, the future might be uncertain. In part this may have been the case. But it was probably deeper than this and was in reality closely connected with that abiding legacy from the past that had been first formulated by Selwyn, Shadwell and Egan. Steve Fairbairn quite early on showed that he was aware of this aspect of the whole issue. Writing in 1912 in *The Field*, he angrily rejected the tone of some of the criticisms of his Jesus crews: 'Jesus takes great offence at being told they are not rowing in the orthodox style, as it implies they are being taught something harmful to rowing, and they feel as if the public looked upon them as being guilty of doing something shady.'[21] It was a significant reaction. In behaving as they did, Fairbairn and those who came under his charge were being made to feel that they were breaking the unwritten code that was at the very heart of the beliefs of the praetorian guard. It was a very serious charge, even if it was only made implicitly, but that it could even be hinted at is enough to explain the depth of feeling aroused on both sides by the controversy. Typical was the view of one, Anthony Haigh, writing in the *Cambridge Review* during November 1928, the occasion being the suggestion that fixed seats should be abolished in the Lent races. He argued that:

> achievement results from a striving after ideals . . . And now the ideals of Cambridge rowing are in the balance. If the proposed reform is rejected, there is still hope, for that will mean that Cambridge oarsmen have not yet lowered their standard. But if it is introduced, then we may know that Cambridge rowing has passed the height of its glory and entered upon its decline. For even if the magnificent successes of the past few years continue for awhile, the art of rowing will be aiming at lower ideals.[22]

Such feelings should not be lightly dismissed. It is not perhaps without significance that the phrase about a man always playing with a straight bat is taken as an indication of his absolute honesty and probity. And the analogy with cricket has a parallel interest. C. B. Fry, amongst the greatest batsmen and athletes of the pre-1914 generation, once wrote that: 'being by nature a rebel, I used to heave a short ball round to the on boundary on slow wickets, even if it was straight. An advantage was that the opposing captain never by any chance put a fieldsman there; he expected you to drive to the off-side like a gentleman.'[23] One cricket historian has argued that before the Great War, years when the amateur batsmen were at their zenith, most were taught and were expected to play to the off-side, the off and cover drives being the delight of the game. It was a risky way of playing the game since the batsmen were always likely to give a catch to the waiting slips and gully, but that was part of the joy of cricket as it was played at that time. A flowing batsman might be unlucky but he was at least giving the bowler a reasonable chance; on the other hand, if he was fortunate, he would construct an innings full of splendid off-side strokes like Fry's gentleman player. The decline of the real amateur after the war and the increasing dominance of the professional player meant that there was a change. The latter could not afford to take such risks, since his contract depended on his getting runs consistently and carefully if he was not to lose his job. He, therefore, set about accumulating runs, steadily and often slowly, not caring too much on which side of the wicket they were scored. But he would tend to eschew the off-side play so beloved of the pre-war amateurs since he could not afford to gamble his career. Many of the old guard, especially P. F. Warner, regretted the changes that were taking place, since they appeared fundamentally to be altering the game. With what appeared to be the disappearance of the correct manner of playing the ball, the Corinthian spirit was apparently disappearing.[24] Edward Lyttelton, a member of a distinguished cricketing family and who was to succeed Warre as headmaster at Eton, once compared the pleasure of composing a fine pentameter to the joy of a good off-drive.[25] But the chance of showing good form in both was something that was confined to very few.

Cricket was, of course, a much larger game with a considerable national following. Nor, as far as rowing was concerned, was there any chance at that time that the professional element would have any influence at all. But that one group within the elite circle might be sowing seeds of corruption was, in itself, worse than any possible professional interference because the charmed group was supposed to share together certain values and methods that were by tradition incorruptible. That there were signs of adulteration was, therefore, tantamount to heresy and betrayal, calling into question the time-honoured code that it had taken almost a century to frame and develop. Hence the almost religious fervour of the antagonists on occasions. But both forgot that over-devout factions generated their own kinds of intolerance and ritual excesses, especially in the hands of the newly converted, zealous often beyond reason. As S. M. Bruce and others had noticed, there were some very odd crews on the Thames, Isis and Cam, supposedly advertising the virtues of their particular fixations.

III

Nevertheless, though some at the time would hardly have agreed, the arguments were basically healthy. As it had established itself, the elite group could easily have fallen into the trap of congratulating itself that all was well in the best of all possible worlds. The almost too comfortable regimes established on the Isis, Cam and the Tideway, with Henley as the common meeting place for the best exponents from each of them, could without too much difficulty have resulted in a situation of mutual complacency that would not have benefited the sport at all. The debate about how to cope with foreign crews and international regattas had had something of this attitude about it and the rejection of the Little England position carried with it the implications that, at some stage, crews from this country would be beaten and that they might be forced to reconsider their particular methods of conducting their affairs.

In the minds of some a degree of degeneration had been obvious since the turn of the century. W. H. Eyre, writing in 1919, lamented what he believed was a decline in the standard of metropolitan rowing. He had no doubt 'the Tideway rowing clubs had a very uphill and ceaseless struggle against the forces of ease and enjoyment which had so insidiously encroached on the battleground of British manliness'.[26] Coming as it did immediately after the Great War, this might seem a little unfair and lacking in generosity but it must be assumed that he was referring to the years before 1914. He was not alone in taking such a lugubrious view. Speaking at the annual dinner of London RC in February 1914, Lord Ampthill, president of the club, former Oxford blue and a man who had once briefly stood-in as the Viceroy of India, regretted that 'no one in these days wants to be subject to moral discipline or any other discipline'.[27] No doubt there were other diversions such as tennis, golf, the bicycle and even the motor car and in the face of them rowing clubs, even such important ones as London RC and Thames RC had to present themselves as something more than just good social meeting places. But taking the high moral ground and condemning the younger generation was not quite the same as arguing about the merits or otherwise of the English orthodox style. But there may well have been a connection. Although the main metropolitan clubs had always been innovators – pioneering the sliding seat and experimenting with the swivel rowlock –

it was easy for them to forget the kind of hard work and toughness that had once characterised some of their earlier, pioneering crews, such as those produced by Thames RC during the late 1870s and early 1880s by Eyre and James Hastie.[28] When a group of enthusiasts did arrive, they sometimes found it a little difficult at first to make any impression on those who preferred to dwell fondly on the past. Such was the four produced in 1907 by Jack Beresford, senior, the father of the famous sculler, that at first had to row as virtually a private combination in a boat that Beresford himself had bought. Possibly the kind of strictures about the state of contemporary youth did not in this case apply since Beresford was in fact forty-two at the time. Accepted by Thames RC, it won the Stewards at Henley in 1909 and 1911 and gained the silver medal for Great Britain in the coxed four event at the 1912 Olympics. To Eyre, remembering perhaps that in his own youth he too had been something of a rebel whom Thames RC had taken some time to appreciate, Beresford's four was a splendid example. Writing of its first victory in the Stewards over the Magdalen four that had won the gold medal at the Olympics the previous year, he commented that: 'the race was won as I like to see a first-class race won – viz. through hard work, constant work, rigid self-denial in training, and iron determination and endurance in the contest'.[29] But this four had triumphed not over the retrograde elements of modern youth – the other three men were youngsters – but over the conservative forces within the club against which it had to prove and justify itself. However gloomy the likes of Eyre and Ampthill might be, they could easily forget that their clubs had once been innovators and that old heresies once accepted could easily turn into forms of orthodoxy that inhibited initiative. Such complacency could very quickly lead to snorts of contemptuous derision at those who suggested a different approach. It was but a short step to accusing the latter of ignoring the straight bat method and therefore of breaking the hallowed code of acceptable behaviour. Beresford's crew had not been afraid to make their point by combining some of the old ways, largely long distance rowing, with some of the new, particularly the use of the swivel rowlock. Their success justified their iconoclastic approach and they became much honoured members of Thames RC. With a group of men of this nature in its midst, it was perhaps not totally surprising that Thames should ask Steve Fairbairn to be the captain immediately after the end of the war. He was to prove highly successful.

The tradition that was established was an enviable one. Seen in terms of Henley alone, Thames RC won the Grand Challenge Cup three times between 1920 and 1939 and were beaten finalists on a further five occasions. In the Stewards, the club had four successes and two further crews reached the final. In 1926, following a disagreement with some members of Thames RC, Fairbairn transferred his attention to London RC. It had taken some years for that club to recover after the war but Fairbairn found that sound foundations had already been laid by R. A. Nisbet, the captain, during 1924–27. Immediately London RC was able to establish its ascendancy again, winning the Grand at Henley four times before 1939 and being the beaten finalist once. It took the Stewards twice and reached the final a further five times. Both clubs also showed considerable strength in depth with a significant number of wins in the other Henley events for which they were qualified as well as producing several international oarsmen.

It is unlikely that all these metropolitan successes can be solely attributed to the presence of Steve Fairbairn. He certainly acted as catalytic agent but in both the clubs there were clear indications that change and some experiment would be welcomed. Beresford's four prior to 1914 had considerably altered the attitudes in Thames RC and, without producing anything quite so effective or dramatic, London RC was in the process of boating some more than competent oarsmen before Fairbairn arrived to coach them. But another explanation for this revival of rowing on the Tideway during the inter-war years – and it was to continue for a few more years after 1945 – was the renewed connection with the universities, more particularly with Cambridge. It was less the number of former blues and good college oarsmen who decided to join them than the emergence once more of the old rivalry at Henley that had been such a strong motivating force during the early years of London RC. In producing crews capable of giving both Leander and the best of the colleges a good race, the metropolitan clubs were not only stimulating the efforts of the universities and the colleges but showing that there was, in fact, no erosion of those attitudes that some members of the orthodox school claimed as their own.

At Cambridge, in spite of fears to the contrary, this had never been the case. The inter-war years were among the most successful enjoyed by that university both in terms of winning the Boat Race more often than not and in enjoying considerable prestige at Henley. The colleges were in fact divided over the Fairbairn and Jesus approach, some adopting it enthusiastically, others treating it with contempt. The Boat Race crews rowed in the main in the orthodox manner but that did not prevent a good many men from the Fairbairn stable gaining their blues. If anything, the presence of such a controversial character in their midst stimulated discussion and certainly forced those who favoured the orthodox approach to ensure that it was done sensibly and effectively. Crises there were on occasions, such as the resignation of the two Cambridge coaches in 1935, but the basic strength was there and a system had emerged that produced not only good university crews but strong college boats as well.

The same was not true of Oxford. In the Boat Race it managed only three victories during the inter-war years. At Henley, the record of Oxford college crews was poor compared with that of Cambridge. The explanations at the time were many. One was a lack of proper interest on the part of the dons, especially their insistence on setting the main examinations so that they interfered with Henley. A Leander member wrote to *The Times* in July 1929 admitting that, although academic matters ought to take precedence, there was surely room for some flexibility: 'As things now are, it would appear the greatest obstacle to the recovery of Oxford rowing is the apathy of the authorities in this matter.'[30] In its spring issue of 1930 the Oxford magazine, *Isis*, discussed the matter, suggesting that the main responsibility must rest with the Oxford coaches, one of whom was G. C. Bourne. He had in fact not looked after an Oxford Boat Race crew since 1927, but his influence and that of his disciples was still there. The hint that someone with new ideas might revive rowing on the Isis carries with it the implication that it was perhaps a pity that no similar figure to Steve Fairbairn existed to jolt the oarsmen out of their malaise. The article thought that at least the idea was worth trying, assuming someone could be found, and that the time might come 'when we shall no longer gauge the magnitude of our victory by the narrowness of our defeat'.[31] It was perhaps a little hard on Bourne, among the most intelligent and innovative of coaches, albeit strictly within the bounds of orthodoxy. In his defence and of those who had been influenced by him, it should be noted that the occasional presence of successful Cambridge coaches at Oxford, Peter Haig-Thomas, F. J. Escombe, K. M. Payne and J. H. Gibbon, did nothing to stop the run of defeats in spite of there being some promising material among the oarsmen.[32] But the fact remains that there was little at Oxford of that obvious excitement that seemed to characterise the Cam. The result was a loss of confidence and belief in the methods being used which the occasional appearance of Fairbairn on the Isis did little to relieve.[33]

IV

In spite of Oxford's woeful record, the standard of all these crews, whether on the metropolitan Thames or from the two universities, whether coached in the orthodox manner or in that of Fairbairn, remained high. They were the best in the country and able to hold their own in the main at international level, although their speed did not much improve over that of the 1890s crews. The record for the Grand Challenge Cup at Henley had been set by Leander in 1891 and equalled by New College, Oxford, six years later. Their time of 6 minutes 51 seconds was only once to be bettered during the inter-war years – by Leander in 1934 in 6 minutes 44 seconds.[34] The situation in the Ladies Challenge Plate, the main event for college eights and school crews, was not very different. Eton had set the record of 6.56 in 1911. It was beaten by one second by Pembroke College, Cambridge in 1921 and improved to 6.48 by Jesus College, Cambridge in 1934. But by and large the times remained similar to those set forty years earlier. One particular record remarkably survived even longer. At the 1911 regatta, the Beresford four had split into two pairs for the Silver Goblets. They dead-heated with each other in the semi-final and their time of 8.08 was not to be beaten until 1952. The most obvious statistic at Henley was the relative failure during these years of Eton College. Between 1864, when the Eton eight first won the Ladies, and 1914, the school won the cup twenty-one times. Between the wars, Eton had only one victory in 1921, although other schools, Shrewsbury in 1932 and Radley in 1938, won the event. The explanation of this decline in fortune, like that at Oxford, is far from clear. The fact that Eton provided, during those same years, more blues at Cambridge than at Oxford might suggest that basically there was not much wrong with the school's rowing and that the apparent decline was simply relative.[35]

Although some international competition had been accepted by the majority of these oarsmen, in some cases with enthusiasm, the world of the elite clubs was still the self-contained one of the last quarter of the previous century. It remained too essentially an exclusive one, insulated from many of the problems that faced the smaller and above all, the provincial clubs. As always, Henley Royal Regatta and the Boat Race were where they advertised their virtues and both received generous coverage in the quality press. The Boat Race remained – and still is – the most lasting legacy of the age of the praetorian guard. A private match between two universities, the last remnant of those private duels that had so characterised the rowing scene in its early days, it is for the public at large the most lasting image of rowing, more important than international competitions and making a far greater impact than the local regatta or even Henley. Normally a somewhat dull affair since the great majority of the races are decided during the first half, the expectations about the Boat Race are probably greater than the actuality. Nevertheless, it remains an important sporting event, broadcast annually since 1927, one of the few occasions when rowing actually engages public attention.[36] That it should do so during the 1920s and 1930s when one university always seemed to win – and has continued to do so during the 1970s and 1980s when the other university has reversed the trend – allows of no simple explanation. In part the answer must lie in the spectacle of two crews of young men publicly allowing themselves to engage in a gladiatorial contest quite unlike any other. They have trained for one day and for one race and few of them will ever become public heroes. As a leading article in *The Times* expressed it just before the 1923 Boat Race, such an oarsman 'seeks a common, not an individual, triumph, and these things will never be without their appeal'.[37] Moreover, he was an amateur, admittedly one who belonged to an exclusive group, open to few to join, but without any hint of duplicity or skulduggery.

It was that aspect of sporting life that was so important for the praetorian guard. There were no doubt unfortunate elements and occasions, not normally malicious in intention, of the kind that inspired the writings of someone like Max Beerbohm. They had been a feature of rowing for years. The antics of W. B. Woodgate during the 1860s stand witness to that, sometimes commendable in their consequences, on others reprehensible.[38] Their apparent division into two antagonistic sects seemed at the time a debilitating drain on their once clear purpose and aim. But, except in the hands of the worst coaches of either camp, the results were to be admired, the fruit of much heart-searching and wrestling, some of it frankly semantic in character. But, as Steve Fairbairn's son once pointed out. 'There is as much to be said against totalitarian *Gleichschaltung* of English rowing as of anything else English. It is not the way of free men; and I have not heard it suggested that anyone has discovered and codified the perfection of rowing. We all have something to learn about rowing whether we call ourselves Fairbairn or Orthodox.'[39] And it may well be that the double series of arguments about international competition and the alternatives to rigid orthodoxy of style did something to break that tight and uncompromising mould that characterised the attitudes of the ARA during the years immediately after the Great War. In many ways, its committee had emerged as the last of the old Bourbons, rather sadly out of touch with that element in its ranks which was capable of producing its best crews. It had the sense not to pronounce on the virtues of this or that way of rowing a boat but it was unfortunate that, on occasions, some of the representatives of orthodoxy could suggest that even to consider alternatives was tantamount to betraying the code of behaviour that in fact they all admired.

Charles Rew, a member of several of the successful Thames RC crews during the early 1920s, once asked Steve Fairbairn on the eve of an important race whether or not he thought they would win. He was startled by the reply: 'I think you will but does it matter, so long as you enjoy your race and do your best?'[40] Such sentiments echoed those expressed earlier by R. C. Lehmann, one of the finest apostles of the orthodox code: 'What, after all, is a sportsman,' he asked,

> As I understand the breed he is one who has not merely braced his muscles and developed his endurance by the exercise of some great sport, but has, in the pursuit of that exercise learnt to control his anger, to be considerate to his fellowmen, to take no mean advantage, to resent as a dishonour the very suspicion of trickery, to bear aloft a cheerful countenance under disappointment, and never to own himself defeated until the last breath is out of his body.[41]

The values of Selwyn, Shadwell and Egan had bitten deep, no matter what the style of rowing might be.

Notes

1 G. Nickalls, *Life's A Pudding, An Autobiography* (London, 1939), p. 213.
2 *Ibid.*, p. 199.
3 David Haig-Thomas, *I Leaped before I Looked, Sport at Home and Abroad* (London, 1936), p. 82.
4 Charles Crawley, *Trinity Hall – The History of a Cambridge College, 1350–1975* (Cambridge, 1977), p. 182.
5 G. C. Bourne, *A Textbook of Oarsmanship* (London, 1925), p. 136.
6 *Ibid.*, p. 374.
7 *Ibid.*, pp. 374–5.
8 R. C. Lehmann, *The Complete Oarsman* (London, 1908), pp. 152–6, 246.
9 G. C. Drinkwater and T. R. B. Saunders, *The University Boat Race – The Official History, 1829–1929* (London, 1929), p. 116.
10 *The Spectator*, 15 June 1907.
11 *The Field*, 20 July 1912 – Letter from W. B. Close.

12 D. C. R. Stuart, Then and now – rowing', the *Badminton Magazine of Sports and Pastimes*, XXXVII, 1913, pp. 10–27.
13 Bourne, *Oarmanship*, p. ix.
14 *Granta*, xxxvi, 25 February 1927, p. 90.
15 *The Times*, 27 January 1933.
16 *Ibid.*, 11 December 1934; S. Fairbairn, *Chats on Rowing* (London, 1934), p. 22; Ian Fairbairn, ed., *Steve Fairbairn on Rowing* (London, 1951), p. 356.
17 Bourne, *Oarmanship*, p. viii.
18 R. D. Burnell, *Swing Together* (London, 1952), p. 59.
19 P. Haig-Thomas and M. A. Nicholson, *The English Style of Rowing* (London, 1958); R. Meldrum, *Rowing and Coaching – Notes on One of the Fine Arts* (London, 1950); *Rowing to a Finish* (London, 1955), *passim*.
20 R. D. Burnell, *The Oxford and Cambridge Boat Race* (London, 1954), pp. 88–9.
21 *The Field*, 13 July 1913.
22 Anthony Haigh, 'The menace to Cambridge rowing', *Cambridge Review*, 2 November 1928.
23 D. Birley, *The Willow Wand – Some Cricket Myths Explored* (London, 1979), p. 17.
24 L. le Quesne, *The Bodyline Controversy* (London, 1983), pp. 132–3, 140–1.
25 J. R. de S. Honey, *Tom Brown's Universe – The Development of the Victorian Public School* (London, 1977), p. 114.
26 T. A. Cook, *Rowing at Henley* (London, 1919), p. xviii.
27 London RC., *From Strength to Strength – 1856–1981: Portrait of London R.C.* (London, 1981), p. 12.
28 W. H. Eyre on Thames RC in R. C. Lehmann, *The Complete Oarsman*, Chapter XVII; on some of the alternatives becoming available to the middle class anxious for exercise – tennis and golf in particular as suburban recreations – see Richard Holt, *Sport and the British – A Modern History* (Oxford, 1989), pp. 350–1.
29 Cook, *Rowing at Henley*, pp. xix-xxi.
30 *The Times*, 6 July 1929.
31 *Isis Magazine*, April 1930.
32 Burnell, *Boat Race*, pp. 86–90.
33 *The Times*, 9 June 1927.
34 Burnell, *Swing Together*, Chapter 2.
35 L. S. R. Byrne and E. L. Churchill, *The Eton Book of the River* (Eton, 1935), pp. 230–4.
36 G. O. Nickalls, *A Rainbow in the Sky* (London, 1974), pp. 151–5.
37 *The Times*, 16 March 1923.
38 W. B. Woodgate, *Reminiscences of an Old Sportsman* (London, 1909), pp. 384–5, where Woodgate relates how on the eve of one of the Boat Races in which he rowed, he organised a meeting between the two crews one evening in which they watched his terrier kill a cat in an enclosed room. The feline corpse apparently floated between the two crews the next day.
39 Ian Fairbairn, *Steve Fairbairn*, p. 39.
40 *Ibid.*, p. 63.
41 *Punch*, 26 June 1907.

6

The difficult years

The temptation to see the ARA and the NARA as rival bodies, touting their goods among the clubs and regattas to increase the strength of one against the other, might seem part of the natural order of things during the inter-war years. In fact neither behaved in quite that way. Before 1939 both found it difficult to command the loyalty of all oarsmen in the country, a good many of whom regarded the two associations with marked indifference. Of the two, the ARA had qualitatively the stronger base and its support along the Thames, Isis and Cam, allowed it to assume a degree of lofty independence that could at times irritate a good number of its own members, especially those in the provinces. The NARA on the other hand had a number of weaknesses that limited its authority and it was forced in 1930 to institute a wholesale reorganisation in an effort to increase its credibility and influence. Meanwhile, clubs and regattas continued to function as circumstances allowed, often without benefit of advice of either association, content to use what were locally inspired organisations that at least understood particular demands and needs.

I

Of the two bodies, the ARA was by the 1920s the larger and more confident, though in some parts of the country its writ was never widely respected or honoured. It had a considerable number of affiliated clubs running up through the Midlands in to the North West but in other parts of the provinces it was consulted on occasion but was otherwise virtually ignored. By structure a somewhat closed group, its committee was nevertheless never quite as authoritarian as some of its members liked to think. Its hand had been forced by its leading oarsmen over the business of international competition which it continued to contemplate for the next twenty years with sulky suspicion. Nor was it over-enthusiastic about becoming involved in the ordinary affairs of the clubs and regattas. It was content to delegate such matters to the various local associations, a situation that was formalised in 1922 when all ARA clubs were arranged as six divisions with representatives on the main central committee. One spokesman recalled that prior to then, 'provincial rowing clubs were a disorganised mess, clubs were organising their own regattas, everybody was treading on other people's corns'.[1] One unforeseen result of this was to strengthen the annual meeting of the provincial committee, insulating the main ARA officials from the clubs and regattas but providing at the same time a useful forum for criticism. But the main ARA committee remained complacently content with the general situation surrounding it. Ignoring the NARA, stuffily suspicious of foreigners and colonials, it left, by a form of indirect rule, the domestic calendar to those who knew most about it. At the time it studiously and rightly refused to become involved in the one issue of the day that threatened to divide its membership, the conflicting and sectarian quarrels over the ideas of Steve Fairbairn, even though in the eyes of some the questioning of the tenets of orthodoxy was akin to treason. Throughout its existing records there is no derogatory reference to Fairbairn or his disciples and it is doubtful whether the issue was ever officially discussed. It would, in fact, have been quite improper if it had been, though for some of the older members of the ARA committee it might at times have seemed the most pressing problem facing English rowing of the day. Fortunately, however, they managed to resist the temptations presented by the issue.

The ARA had one distinct advantage over the NARA. When in 1894 it decided on an exact definition of a professional, it not only defeated its own diehards but appeared to give the NARA largely what it had wanted three years earlier. But, whether by accident or design, Lehmann's strategem allowed ARA clubs to admit as members many who were obvious candidates for the NARA. Often, therefore, the two associations were in competition and this must have seriously limited the NARA's field for manoeuvre. The situation was exacerbated further by the NARA's very proper determination to avoid any hint that its members were not amateurs. In 1895 it rejected the idea of a paid secretary 'as it might lead to the thin edge of the wedge of professionalism'.[2] In the same year and for the same reasons it refused to accept the claims of a lighterman and his apprentice to be considered as amateurs.[3] However genuine the motives of such men, the NARA could not afford to give itself as a hostage to fortune. The result was that there were occasions when its judgement could seem unnecessarily punctilious. During 1900 the committee had before it the case of a young man anxious to join one of the clubs on the Lea. Already a member of the Amateur Boxing Association, he worked as a barman, occasionally ferrying customers across the river. Whatever fares he took were immediately given to the publican. The NARA was in no doubt that such conduct made him a professional and that he was totally unacceptable as an amateur.[4]

It was hardly surprising, given such fastidious discrimination, that the NARA committee could, in 1904, lament its relatively small numbers and regret that its name and work were not better known, especially in the provinces.[5] It was in danger at best of getting lukewarm support or, rather worse, of condemning a number of would-be amateurs to the wilderness of rowing through the strictness of its rulings. It was not quite the outcome that had been envisaged by Dr Furnivall.

The first of these alternatives – an unenthusiastic recognition – was the case among the Oxford city clubs. Following the small entry at the Oxford Royal Regatta in 1895, the *Oxford Chronicle* complained that the reason was 'the imposition of unnecessary restrictions as to what constitutes an amateur'.[6] Irritation of that kind could quite easily be aimed at both the associations but, among the local clubs along the Isis, it might have been expected that the NARA would find some sympathy. In fact only one club, the Falcon RC, joined at the onset and then equally quickly allowed its membership to lapse.[7] None of the other Oxford City clubs had joined before 1914 and each must have doubted whether there was any point in doing so. Similar reactions were to be found in other parts of the country. By 1911 in fact, only seven clubs outside the Thames and the Lea had bothered to affiliate to the NARA.[8] One of them, York City, had a few years earlier been in such a parlous state that its secretary had been forced to find the annual subscription out of his own pocket.[9] Before and after the Great War, a number of local associations had emerged, some dating from the 1890s. Although accepting the general tenor of the NARA's code of practice, they resisted the idea of direct affiliation. As well as the group at Oxford, there were others from Hampshire and Dorset, the Midlands and the West of England, while some of the Kent and Sussex coastal clubs viewed the NARA with hesitant and distant interest.[10]

At least where such associations and clubs existed, amateur oarsmen could find some possibility of organised sport and pleasure. But elsewhere the position was more difficult. Two NARA clubs at Jarrow seem by the 1920s to have disappeared. Elsewhere in that area the other amateur clubs remained unaffiliated and their attitudes on the amateur issue were ambivalent, Tyne ARC taking a hard line approach, the two Tees clubs being uncertain. The only alternative, if an oarsman was unacceptable to any of them, was to join one of the many professional clubs in the North East. Each of them had a strong sense of working-class pride and solidarity and on the whole they were not clubs for outsiders. Nor were the financial rewards very great, what there was being earned mainly at the annual fours handicap at Durham Regatta and at the Christmas Handicap for scullers on the Tyne. A similar situation existed on the Thames, primarily at Barnes where the Tradesmen's Rowing Clubs Association had a somewhat ambiguous existence. Already functioning by the late 1880s, it seems likely that it was the final resting place for those who did not easily fit into the NARA's often draconian interpretation of its own rules.[11] By the mid-1920s, however, the TRCA's exact role was becoming a matter of debate. Weybridge RC, for example, had joined the NARA in 1924 and yet it continued to be listed in the TRCA.[12] This may perhaps explain why Charles Tugwell, secretary to the NARA and normally well supplied with accurate information, thought that TRCA oarsmen were amateurs. He was quickly disabused when it was pointed out that Ernest Barry, five times professional sculling champion of the world, was also a member. But it transpired that the TRCA was not itself absolutely certain what it was or what it should be. By 1927 it was trying to distinguish between a genuine professional, such as Barry, and those who were simply on the fringe of the organisation. E. H. Wall of the Thames branch of the NARA claimed to have direct knowledge of the situation since some of his own clubs shared the boat-house at Barnes with the TRCA. He had no doubt that it was a base for professionals but that it was attempting without much success to change its image. He claimed that they 'will accept anybody so long as he has not competed for a staked bet over a certain amount and the trouble is that they cannot agree on the amount'.[13] By the late 1920s, the TRCA seemed to be sorting out its affairs and the committee of the Tideway Boxing Day Charity Regatta made it clear that it would welcome an event under its particular rules.[14] It was in the process of gaining some respectability and that was just as well since, although in a minor key, the TRCA was sounding a note critical of the NARA not being the all-embracing and tolerant body it had originally set out to be.

The situation, therefore, facing the NARA during these post-war years was hardly a satisfactory one. It had not developed as its founders had hoped and it could hardly claim to be a representative body. It had been rudely rebuffed by the Henley stewards in 1919 and had been shabbily treated by the ARA over the Olympic issue. At least, as far as the latter was concerned, it had salvaged some of its pride when an NARA club, Weybridge, provided the coxed four at the 1924 games.[15] But, even over that, the NARA could claim little real credit. Three years earlier, the Weybridge committee could see no point in joining the Thames branch of the NARA and its decision to do so in 1924 seems largely to have been a device to ensure Olympic selection in an event that the ARA totally ignored.[16] As it was, the Weybridge four owed its main debt in terms of advice and training to a number of sympathetic ARA coaches, one of them being Steve Fairbairn.[17] The impression remains that the NARA exercised little real authority. Only along the Lea and parts of the Thames did it have any form of control and even then, as in the case of the Weybridge four, it had not the depth of experience and expertise to be able to offer competent assistance.

II

It was Charles Tugwell, from his vantage as secretary to the NARA, who seems to have been more conscious than some others of the kind of problems facing his association. He was a man of considerable sense and much ingenuity. The NARA and indeed rowing as a sport was to owe him a considerable debt, comparable to that previously exercised in the ARA by Lehmann. It was Tugwell who organised three conferences in London during 1927–9 that brought together for the first time all the disparate elements that had some sympathy for the NARA's cause but as yet little real loyalty to it as a governing body. In addition to representatives from the main committee and its two branches on the Lea and the Thames, there were delegates from the Coast ARA, the West of England ARA, the Hampshire and Dorset ARA, Oxford Town Rowing, Norwich, Ipswich and the Cambridgeshire RA. Although the chair was taken by Prebendary P.S.G. Probert, one of the original founders of the NARA, the guiding influence was that of Tugwell.

He had already begun to show a flexible and sensible approach to some of the problems of rules, modifying the over harsh implications of some earlier decisions. Shortly before the first conference in 1927, he had, for example, argued that metropolitan policemen 'who had to use motor-boats in the course of their duty did not violate their status . . . We took the risk of interpreting the rule we have in the spirit rather than in the letter.'[18] The delegates were clearly delighted at such a liberal approach. They did, however, take longer to digest another of his suggestions when it was revealed that, at West Country regattas, the prizes were normally in cash, given to the winning club rather than to the individuals concerned. Such a practice seemed to offend one of the earliest decisions taken by the NARA and raised again the spectre of professionalism.[19] A West Country delegate defended the arrangements as: 'the very existence of our Association and clubs and it is very satisfactory to the regattas. They get the entries and the clubs each get something to help their expenses.' However a good many of those present at the 1927 conference were thrown into confusion by these revelations. But Tugwell, aware that throughout the country there were a good many different conventions and considerable width in the inter-pretation of rules, was ready to place his own gloss on such practices:

> My own personal opinion is that your clubs, by competing with no prospect of immediate personal gain, are more nearly akin to real amateurism than those who compete for a trophy and prizes; for while a crew in the latter case winning would be certain of prizes, a winning crew in your case would get nothing beyond the honour of winning unless their club could afford, at the end of the year, to present them with medals or some such token.

This attempt to reconcile the values of Selwyn, Shadwell and Egan with those of the professionals was almost too much for many of those present until Tugwell, with a final flourish, produced the rules of the New Zealand ARA that allowed precisely the practice common in the West Country.[20]

Tugwell's aim seems to have been to persuade the delegates that there was much merit in diversity and in accepting a liberal and sensible approach to the question of rules. An acceptance of varying the different conventions would lead to a much stronger association, one more attuned to the times and above all capable of growth. During the three conferences, for example, it emerged that there were considerable differences of approach towards those involved in building boats. As one speaker, anxious to support as wide an interpretation as possible, put it: 'There is no logical reason why a man who is practically a carpenter and joiner, who can be put on a rowing boat or on the internal fittings of a liner or on building a battleship, and whose work does not take him into boats to row them about, should be barred.'[21] In the end the delegates basically confirmed the existing NARA definition of an amateur but, when it came to the point about boat-builders, they were allowed to use their discretion and local interpretations were allowed, precisely the approach that Tugwell wished to encourage.

The fundamental issue, however, that was basic to all three conferences was the need to set up 'a central body for the purpose of controlling amateur rowing'.[22] Once the problems of local conventions and usages had been resolved, the larger one was more easy to solve. It was agreed that the NARA should be reformed as from 1 January 1930 as a limited company and that the affiliated associations should be 'given power to make such rules and by-laws as local conditions make expedient provided they do not infringe any of the rules of the N.A.R.A.'[23] It was a satisfactory compromise, allowing a modicum of control to run parallel with a fairly wide degree of tolerance in a much more widely-based organisation. Each of the associations was asked to discuss the proposals and in some areas the debate was a vigorous one. At club level there was some suspicion. Exeter ARC at its committee meeting in March 1929 urged the delegates to the final conference to keep both an open and a wary mind. It expressed particular concern that the right of the West of England ARA to allow money prizes should be preserved and so great was its alarm on the point that one member 'wondered what would be gained by the W.E.A.R.A. becoming part of, and subservient to, the proposed larger organisation'.[24]

These were proper questions to ask and only time and experience would provide an answer to them. But as long as Charles Tugwell was secretary, showing his usual tact and sense, the new arrangements seemed workable. A coherent body was being set up that recognised the need for some form of central control but which was able to tolerate differences of approach. It was a pragmatic solution that took into account local variations and practices by encouraging a degree of diversity. At last the NARA seemed in a position to reflect the larger vision that had inspired its founders during the early 1890s.[25]

III

While the two main associations were setting their houses into some form of order, clubs throughout the country tried with varying degrees of success to carry on with their business. It would have been something of a disappointment to the respective secretaries of both associations had they realised how seldom their organisations were referred to in club and regatta minute books. Until after the Second World War, the number of unaffiliated clubs was large, especially so in the North East. Although the ARA had given its blessing to the reconstituted Northern Rowing Council in 1926, neither had very much authority and they were unable, for example, to prevent Durham Regatta imposing its own local rules when its committee saw fit.[26] Although causing some irritation, the arrangements seemed to work reasonably well and there was no obvious cause to change them. In 1926 the provincial committee of the ARA suggested that gentle hints might be dropped to the unaffiliated clubs and regattas, recommending the benefits of membership.[27] Little was in fact done perhaps because it was not all that obvious what they were. In any case such a suggestion lacked some degree of conviction when, two years later, the same body could record its view that 'there is a great cleavage between the Thames and the provinces'.[28] The reality was at that time that there was a qualitative difference in standard between most provincial crews and the best metropolitan and college boats. The sympathy and interest of most members of the ARA committee lay with the latter. But, in any case, it must be questioned whether the provincial clubs would have welcomed more interference and direction from the centre or whether the ARA or the NARA could often have made any useful contribution. When, in 1933, Kingston RC from Hull suggested that a loan-fund might be set up under the ARA, the annual meeting of the provincial committee dismissed the idea as not being part of the business of governing associations.[29] Not until the advent of the National Fitness Campaign just before the Second World War was a mechanism found to direct funds towards clubs with needs of that kind.

During the inter-war years, the effects of the depression and an uncertain future made life far from comfortable for many clubs and regattas. The annual report of the NARA for 1931, for example, stated that: 'the unemployment rife throughout the country, the heavier taxation, the salary and wage cuts, the economy that has been made necessary by these and other causes – all have contributed to make the past year one of great anxiety.'[30] But what these difficult years also revealed was the fundamental frailty of structure of much English rowing, the consequence of almost too rapid a growth during the last quarter or so of the previous century. These were problems that neither the ARA nor the NARA were equipped to solve and clubs were, as a result, thrown onto their own often slender resources, finding answers to each crisis as best they could.

Those that survived best were the select group of metropolitan-based clubs, those that had earlier forged the crucial link with Oxford and

Cambridge, and which were powerful in the inner councils of the ARA. Occasionally even clubs of this kind could temporarily stumble. Kingston RC on the Thames was faced in 1934 with a worrying financial situation and a demand from their landlord for an increase in rent. The answer was found in better control and management when they moved the next year to a different site on rather better terms.[31] But for the most part, such clubs used rather different criteria for judging a successful year from the majority. In 1932, the captain of London RC could gloomily report on what he called 'a year of defeat', one in which the Thames Cup and the Wyfolds had been won at Henley.[32] Such luxurious melancholy was rarely afforded to most of the smaller and less-favoured clubs throughout the country. Occasionally they might enjoy the excitement of a Henley victory – Burton in 1902, Birmingham in 1904, Royal Chester in 1891 and 1924, Reading RC in 1934 and 1935, all in the Wyfolds – but for the most part a good year would be judged by a few wins at local regattas, a modest balance on the revenue account and a fresh coat of paint on the boat-house door. They faced problems unlikely to occur at the larger metropolitan clubs, however much the latter might groan at only two Henley wins in a season.

Clubs such as London RC, Thames RC and Leander had two advantages that normally insulated them against some of the worst kind of difficulties. One was their size, large enough to embrace an active group of oarsmen as well as others to whom membership was largely a matter of social prestige and pride. The second was the ownership of their sites which meant that they were not dependent on the changing whims of landlords. Both London RC and Thames RC, once they had established themselves, set up limited companies separate from the clubs themselves but in which members were encouraged to buy shares. By this means both were able to purchase the lease and the land on which they then built their boat-houses.[33] But the many clubs set up during the 1860s and 1870s were unable to arrange matters quite so carefully. Liverpool Victoria tried a variation of this plan during the 1890s when the expansion of the Mersey Docks and Harbour Board forced the club to seek a new site. A small company was floated with £1 shares but only to finance the construction of the boat-house since the lease was not for sale. After 1920, the Harbour Board again moved the club to another location, although careful to find them a piece of land large enough for their needs. Although the new tenancy was only a monthly one, Liverpool Victoria found the £700 for the new building by once more issuing £1 bonds. The result was that by 1934, 400 of them still remained as one of the club's liabilities.[34]

One consequence of such tenancy agreements was that clubs could be inhibited both in terms of their activities and in effecting necessary repairs. Because the Harbour Board had initially given Liverpool Victoria only a small site, the committee was forced, just before 1914, to hive off the pleasure boat section elsewhere, thus effectively cutting the club into two.[35] Weybridge RC during the 1920s anxiously wished to repair and extend their boat-house but was rightly cautious since the tenancy was only for a year at a time. Attempts to alter it met with no success, the landlord assuring them that he would neither increase the rent nor bother them in any way. Such protestations, however, did not prevent him from presenting the highest tender for repairing the boat-house.[36] The effect of such unstable tenancies in upsetting a club's normal routine could be considerable, as happened to Middlesbrough ABC at the turn of the century. Quite unexpectedly, in the middle of the 1900 rowing season, the landlord announced that he would need the site within two months to allow him to expand his factory space. Boats had to be moved, temporary storage found, frantic searching for an alternative piece of land begun, and discussions entered into about what the new boat-house would be like and how much the club could afford. The best would have been an old cycle shed that would have to be transported in pieces but it proved too costly. In the end the landlord relented, granting the club an adjacent piece of ground but still necessitating a new building. The total effect of all this was effectively to disrupt two season's rowing.[37]

Size of membership proved a difficult and uneasy problem. On a good many rivers, there were simply too many rowing clubs, the consequence in the main of the enthusiasm of the late nineteenth century. On the Tees there were two with a small professional club in attendance. On the Tyne, in addition to the professional groups, there were Tyne ARC, South Shields, Mid-Tyne, Jarrow and Tynemouth, with Newcastle RC, Northern RC and Ryton RC having already disappeared before the Great War. On the Trent at Nottingham there were five clubs just before 1914, while the West Country between the wars gave an embarrassingly wide choice. A relatively small place like Bideford had two, the Dart club at Totnes was close to Dartmouth ARC, while the Exe from 1927 had Exeter ARC, the older, and Port Royal ARC, the successor to St Thomas RC that had ceased in 1921. What was interesting about these West Country arrangements was that, while all competed under NARA and West of England ARA rules, several emphasised delicate social distinctions as far as membership was concerned. Exeter ARC, for example, had a distinct middle-class quality about it, while the rival Port Royal was largely working-class.[38] Intense local rivalry meant that the individual identity of a club tended to be preserved at almost any cost. Nevertheless, there had always been some amalgamations as the less viable struggled to survive. At Worcester, nine clubs that had existed during the 1860s and 1870s had been reduced to the single Worcester RC by the 1880s.[39] Agecroft RC on the Irwell was to be the beneficiary as several clubs along that river closed just before and after the Great War.[40] Walton RC amalgamated with the short-lived Oatlands RC in 1934, while the Tees ABC contemplated a similar approach to Middlesbrough ABC in 1932, only to recognise the sense of such a move in 1946.[41] A similar solution was found in the West Country when the two Exeter clubs joined together just after the Second World War.[42]

There seemed no common set of solutions to the problem of membership, not least because there was an increasing list of alternative possibilities such as golf, tennis, cycling and the motor car. By the 1930s, the latter seemed to the Stratford-upon-Avon committee to have become a major obstacle to progress, one member commenting in 1937, that 'many people nowadays had cars and preferred the countryside to the river'.[43] One possible solution was to try to absorb some of these competing activities. As early as 1882, the Stratford club had invited a member of the local bicycle club to join its committee and three years later itself became part of the Midland Counties Athletic Association.[44] Such ventures did not always work. Durham ARC failed in 1891 to set up an athletic section in conjunction with the cricket and tennis clubs, while, four years later, the two Tees clubs did manage to combine for a similar purpose only to find that the costs were too high.[45] Forming an alliance with a local swimming group could prove more fruitful. Both Exeter and Weybridge during the 1920s established fairly strong links in that way, discovering that the costs were relatively low and that swimming introduced some degree of variety into their annual regattas.[46] Evesham RC tried, during the inter-war years, to continue its tradition of appealing to a wide membership but found, in part because of some heavy losses on its regattas, that financial problems forced it into often contradictory decisions. In 1930, unable to afford the cost of maintaining the club punts, the committee sold them and yet, four years later, it was urging the need to advertise itself as a club in the widest sense, anxious to encourage those wishing to use the pleasure boats, play tennis and go into the gymnasium.[47] Its near neighbour at Stratford found itself during the 1930s faced not just with a falling membership but with a large deficit, exacerbated by an extension to the boat-house.[48] But the answer was not in this case to try to widen the membership. On the contrary, equipment was sold and it was this dilemma that led to the acrimonious debate that effectively killed off the pleasure boating activities of the club.[49] Exeter ARC had been forced into a similar decision as early as 1928 for the same reason – expense.[50] The long-standing argument between the competitive and the boating elements was effectively brought to an end by such financial problems. But there were obvious dangers in such conclusions, not least that a club would lose something of its attractiveness to the community of which it was a part. Matters were made a great deal worse when the quarrels were given a public airing in the press, as happened at Stratford.

Most committees, nevertheless, tried to find the answer to their problems by increasing numbers in their clubs. But, as Liverpool Victoria had discovered before 1914, too large a membership on a limited site simply uncovered a different set of problems. A small selection of boats, even when numbers were modest, obviously limited the amount of rowing, as happened at Wansbeck where for a time outings were limited to a mere twenty minutes.[51] Some of the NARA clubs, such as those at Oxford and on the Lea, may well have found the most sensible solution to the problem. Few of them could afford equipment of their own and they, therefore, established their headquarters with local boat-builders from whom they rented boats on a seasonal basis. The Falcon RC at Oxford hired its craft from Salter or Talboy, a system that worked well for many years, the club not owning a boat of its own until 1949.[52]

This was not, however, an alternative open to most clubs whose committees therefore were faced with the delicate task of ensuring sufficient members to balance the books with an adequate pool of boats to satisfy most needs. Occasionally a club was able to solve the equation. In the years immediately after the Great War, Tees ABC found itself forced to limit numbers by introducing a waiting list but, as the recession began to be felt in the area, numbers very quickly began to fall.[53] Derby RC had 120 members in 1923 and recruitment and the financial state of the club remained reasonably healthy until 1939. It in fact benefited from its long tradition of drawing a significant part of its membership from the Midland Railway Company which was able to weather the vicissitudes of the time rather better than some industries.[54] Different local circumstances, however, particularly those in the North East during the 1920s and 1930s, could discourage even the most active club committee, especially if its own perception of itself was a further handicap. Tyne ARC, for example, although unaffiliated, saw itself firmly in the ARA camp. Possibly because it was so far out of the main stream of events, it could conceive its future, somewhat forlornly, in terms that would have delighted the framers of the 1878 Putney rules but which sadly limited the kind of men who might be welcome in the clubhouse. In 1928, its committee could see the only way forward being to write 'to suitable public schools, varsities, rugby clubs and military garrisons'.[55]

But in one particular the Tyne committee was right. A direct appeal to schools could, if successful, be seen as an investment in the future. It was not a new idea. Derwent RC had benefited from allowing the boys of Derby Grammar School to row from their clubhouse for a quarter of a century until, in the 1880s, a new headmaster had different ideas. But, during the 1930s, the connection was revived, although on the second occasion the school allied itself to Derby RC, gently bolstering an already successful club.[56] After the Great War, Liverpool Victoria allowed the boys of Wallasey Grammar School to become junior members and their presence was the salvation of the club.[57] Tyne itself began to cultivate the Royal Grammar School at Newcastle during the mid-1930s, while Evesham RC did the same with the local grammar school to the immediate benefit of its regatta.[58] Such an arrangement, however, had its dangers. One reason for the closure of Nemesis RC in Manchester just before the Great War was its over-great dependence on the boys of Manchester Grammar School who were stopped from rowing when the High Master became alarmed about the pollution of the river and the large amount of river traffic.[59] There were other risks as well. Exeter ARC had normally recruited its coxes from interested schoolboys but a warning from the local education office that the club was transgressing by-laws led to a hurried inquiry. There seemed no doubt that it was abetting truancy.[60]

There was another source of recruitment but one that was never successfully tapped until after 1945. Women had started to row seriously before the Great War but only in small numbers. The Cecil Ladies BC on the Lea existed before 1914, as did the Furnivall Sculling Club at Hammersmith, founded in 1895 originally for women only. Ross RC had raised the matter of a women's section with the ARA in 1905 but had received no encouragement.[61] Durham ARC received a similar answer in 1913 but had in any case decided against such a project for lack of suitable facilities.[62] Derwent RC had allowed a ladies section in 1907 as long as those concerned boated elsewhere and hired their own craft.

With such lukewarm support, it quickly folded up.[63] The occasional appearance of females at regattas often resembled the side-shows that were largely intended to attract a larger crowd. Wargrave continued to organise races for women and also for mixed crews beyond the turn of the century, while Evesham Regatta in 1909 had a women's coxed sculling race, the prize being a sewing machine.[64]

By the 1920s, however, women's rowing was becoming more active, especially on the Thames. Neither the ARA, nor the NARA, took any real interest in such goings on and in 1923 the Women's ARA was established.[65] It did not always give the best of impressions. The Furnivall Scullers, who might have been expected to be sympathetic, decided in 1925 'that for the time being we withold affiliation to the W.A.R.A. The committee wish to record our dissatisfaction with the management of the association, specifically to the fact that we understand the honorary secretary was party to a professional engaging in a women's race under the association's rules.'[66] The only possible explanation to this bewildering reservation is that the offending woman was a member of Weybridge RC, one of the few clubs with a women's section but also during the immediate post-war period connected to the Tradesmen's Association. But, in a male dominated sport, accusations of this kind quickly ran along the tow-paths and reinforced prejudices against the acceptance of women. The result was that the WARA had to develop quietly on its own. By the 1930s, the Civil Service Ladies had their own boat-house but most of the women's clubs, including those connected with the University of London, used part of Green's Boatyard adjacent to Barnes Bridge.[67] For the moment, at any rate, an influx of women, except at a small number of clubs, was not seen as an acceptable solution to the membership problem. Prejudice had to be overcome and that was going to take time. When, in 1950, Exeter decided to admit women, the chairman grumpily concluded the debate by hoping it would not only be an experiment but a short-lived one at that.[68]

Given many of these problems – low membership, uncertain tenancies, delapidated boat-houses and elderly equipment – it was no wonder that clubs could occasionally become prey to melancholy. At a general meeting of the Tees club in January 1925, it was agreed that 'the club was going down' and that there was 'no demand for a regatta on the River Tees by either spectators or rowing people of other clubs'.[69] Had the committee known at the time that the club possessed seven bow-side blades and only one stroke-side to match, its grief might have been inconsolable.[70] And yet, had it not been for human frailty, some of the problems facing many of the clubs could have been alleviated. A constant and indeed tedious theme in so many minute books was the inability of club officials to persuade members to pay their dues. It was an old problem. The financial statement of the Middlesbrough ABC for 1901–2 was typical. Out of the total annual receipts of £28 12s 10d, £6 2s 6d represented ordinary subscriptions. On the asset side, £6 6s 0d was the amount of subscription arrears. In short, over half the active rowing members were still in debt to the club at the end of the financial year.[71] Figures of this nature were common across the land. Club committees had considered various ways of dealing with the difficulty. Before 1914, some, including Durham ARC, Evesham RC and Furnivall Scullers, were prepared to threaten legal action, so serious was the offence considered.[72] In a few cases, the arrears were so large and numerous that to have brought even a fraction of the offenders before the County courts would have been the most unfortunate of advertisements. In September 1899, for example, Nottingham RC was still owed over one hundred subscriptions.[73] The Tyne ARC committee took a more scrupulous approach, refusing to allow a man to resign instead of paying his subscription on the ground that he would compromise those who had proposed and seconded him.[74] But most clubs, like Evesham, ignored such niceties, preferring to list miscreants on the notice-board and finally expelling those who refused to pay.[75] It was altogether an irritating business, often causing considerable tension, forcing the frustrated chairman of the Stratford club on one occasion to complain that 'from a great many members we have had nothing but trouble in trying to get their subscriptions'.[76]

All these problems were worrying and in some cases they were serious, but their effects were uneven. Clubs in the North East probably felt the most deprived and most vulnerable, while those in the Thames area were more easily able to survive. Significantly, the annual reports of the provincial ARA clubs hardly ever dwell on financial matters and allied difficulties, while the NARA conferences, leading to the 1930 reorganisation, largely ignored such questions in what were fairly wide-ranging debates. Some clubs did in fact collapse but not always for the obvious reasons. Warwick BC, for example, resigned from the ARA in 1926 and stopped competitive rowing simply because there were so many pleasure boats on its particular stretch of the river.[77] But the survival of the fittest had long been part of rowing's history and the strong were only too willing to absorb the weak or to seek a viable alternative by amalgamation.

IV

At the highest level, crews from this country were able to maintain an enviably high standard with no hint that there were underlying difficulties. British crews, for example, were second in the Olympic table of medals during 1900–48 (Table VII). Most of the oarsmen were drawn from the ranks of the praetorian guard and some of them, such as Jack Beresford, proved to be outstanding athletes.[78] Admittedly the pace of the best crews, taking Henley as the main indicator, improved hardly at all during the first half of the century, rarely bettering the times achieved during the late 1880s and the 1890s.[79] But this was hardly a matter of great concern since the oarsmen involved more than held their own at international level.

Table VII, *Olympic rowing medals, 1900–48*

	Gold	Silver	Bronze	Total
USA	19	9	9	37
Great Britain	14	11	2	27
Germany	9	3	5	17
Switzerland	4	4	5	13
Italy	3	7	5	15
Australia	3	–	–	3
France	2	3	2	7
Belgium	1	4	–	5
Denmark	1	3	1	5
Holland	1	1	–	2
Canada	–	1	1	2
Norway	–	–	1	1

Notes
(a) Great Britain did not officially take part in the Olympic Regatta until 1908. George St Ashe, apparently a private entry, won the sculling bronze in 1900.
(b) The USA did not take part in the 1908 and 1912 Regattas while that of 1904 at St Louis in the United States was almost a private American affair, no European nations sending crews.
(c) Germany was not represented at the 1924, 1928 and 1948 Regattas.
(d) Prior to 1920, multiple entries from each nation concerned were allowed in all events.

What is less easy to judge is the quality of rowing outside the main metropolitan clubs and the two universities. Again, just as clubs had responded differently to hard times, so they reacted unevenly when it came to their rowing. Weybridge had produced the Olympic coxed four in 1924 and Nottingham and Union did the same four years later.[80] In

1936 an NARA sculler only lost to his ARA rival by a bare length in a trial for the Olympic team.[81] But, when G. P. Merifield, cox of the victorious Oxford crews of 1937 and 1938, went to Newcastle as a journalist, he was far from impressed by the rowing in the area: 'I have seen crews on the Tyne,' he wrote, 'which have given me the impression of a Bank holiday boating party on the Serpentine rather than that of a club crew out for a training row.'[82] But such a harsh judgement was not surprising, performance on the water in the North East reflecting the general hardships that all the clubs were facing.

Elsewhere, however, more vigour and enterprise were evident. Although in 1901 the chairman of Derby RC had advised against rowing away from home since it might cause some disharmony in the club, his advice fortunately had been forgotten by the 1920s. A reasonably healthy financial situation and a sufficient number of members meant that by the end of the decade Derby was able to embark on a series of successful seasons, including winning the West of England Vase in 1928, one of the most prized of provincial cups. Such was the club's confidence that it entered for the Head of the River Race on the Thames and won the first Head of the Trent in 1935.[83] Agecroft was another that showed commendable initiative, before 1914 sending crews to Evesham and Lancaster and, during the inter-war years, widening its scope still further to include York, Worcester, Derby and Nottingham as well as an occasional appearance at Henley. This admirable approach led to invitations to go abroad, Agecroft rowing in Norway in 1911 and at Hamburg in 1924.[84] These were brave ventures on the part of a provincial club even though they paled into some insignificance compared with London RC, whose oarsmen seemed able to organise races overseas almost at will.[85]

All this kind of activity, especially during the far from easy inter-war years, suggests a degree of resilience in many places that counteracts the prevalent gloom of many club minute books. There were some inhibiting elements, especially the difficulties of transporting boats over even quite short distances. Railways, in theory, had widened oarsmen's horizons but only if they could afford the often high costs. It was an issue that occasionally attracted the ARA's attention. In 1906 its committee decided that it would be unwise to encourage regattas to make a contribution towards the cartage of boats, suggesting that the alternative was to reduce entry fees.[86] Four years later, the ARA wrote to all the main railway companies since travel and carriage 'constitute a heavy burden and so tend to diminish the number of crews entering at a regatta'. It was to no avail since the railways felt they were already being generous by allowing rebates if the crew travelled on the same train as the boat.[87] In 1926 the provincial ARA meeting described the issue as having been 'the bugbear of senior rowing in the provinces for years'.[88] Nor had there been any real improvement two years later. Its meeting was told that the LMS had agreed to treat oars as hand luggage, which must have pleased other passengers in the compartment, but it was far from certain that the other companies would follow suit.[89] The Agecroft representative objected to the unfair treatment of oarsmen since the railways would not recognise regattas as qualifying for concessionary fares in the same way as football matches.[90] In fact a solution did exist since various clubs had been experimenting with specially designed superstructures that could be fitted to lorries.[91] The internal combustion engine was to be an important liberating element for many clubs throughout the country, a more effective agent for change than even the railway train, useful as that had been in its time.

This was but one symptom of changing attitudes as the economic climate of the 1930s showed some signs of improvement. Not all were able to grasp the new opportunities. In the North East, especially, where the effects of the depressions lingered on, the clubs there remained caught in the cumulative misery of the years. Even in areas enjoying some prosperity, a few clubs such as Stratford, unable quite to solve the problems facing them, continued to view the future uneasily. One fundamental issue that was common to a good many clubs was the inevitable tensions between those who wanted some degree of change and those, normally senior members, who saw themselves as the guardians of custom and tradition. During times of stringency the possibility of experimenting was usually avoided. Caution was the obvious course, reinforced among the ARA clubs especially by the somewhat conservative attitudes of its main committee. It was one of the virtues of Steve Fairbairn that his inconclastic approach to rowing a boat, expressed in eccentrically written books and articles, at least made people look at the sport with a fresh mind. Not that too much credit should be given to him since his claims on his own behalf were at times so outrageous as to be self-defeating.[92] Nevertheless, the fact that he could arouse so much controversy was healthy since inevitably some began to question accepted usages and customs.

One apparently unalterable rule was that rowing was essentially a summer sport, clubs opening in the spring and closing at the onset of autumn. Outside Oxford and Cambridge, there were few clubs that departed from this norm until after the 1920s and even after the Second

World War it remained a common practice. Among the first to break it were clubs on the Thames, among which some belonging to the NARA were prominent. The Tideway Boxing Day Charity Regatta began in 1922 and was deliberately designed to attract all sorts and conditions of men. There were scratch coxswainless fours from some of the ARA clubs and, after 1929, some races under Tradesmen's rules. But the major event was the Lord Desborough Cup for eights between the Lea and the Thames branches of the NARA. Following the 1930 reorganisation, all NARA associations could send a representative crew and it was moved to the Interim Regatta in November but remained closely associated with the Boxing Day event.[93] The prospects of taking part in a regatta of this kind encouraged Weybridge RC, for example, to introduce winter training in 1923, including physical exercises as well as rowing. One consequence of all this was that the club produced an Olympic four the next summer.[94] By the early 1930s, the Thames branch of the NARA was further developing such habits by organising a series of winter league races.[95] In the provinces, apart from those involved in the professional Christmas Handicap on the Tyne, the move towards rowing all the year round was less obvious. While Nottingham RC had allowed some winter practice from as early as 1909, Tees ABC confirmed in 1921 its strict rule that the boat-house must close in the autumn of each year.[96]

The most important impetus to winter training on the Thames came from Steve Fairbairn. As coach first of Thames RC and then of London RC, he had encouraged rowing throughout the closed season to counter the apparent advantage of the university college crews.[97] It was largely his idea to begin an annual long-distance, time-trial from Mortlake to Putney to give some point to this winter work. The first Head of the River Race was held in December 1926, with the second not long afterwards in March 1927. The effect on the Tideway was immediate. J. T. Phelps, the old waterman, claimed he had never seen so many eights at work during the winter months, while the editor of the London RC *Report* had no doubt 'that the remarkable advance in both quality and quantity of metropolitan rowing is directly traceable to the influence of this race and Mr. Fairbairn's inspiration'.[98] London RC reacted immediately to all this by innovative methods of training. By the late 1920s, its best oarsmen were expected to train twice a week between October and Easter, the emphasis being on skipping, weight-lifting and rope-climbing, together with long rows on the river during the week-ends.[99] Gradually this idea of long-distance races as the culmination of the winter season began to be accepted. By the 1930s, the NARA had its own Head of the River on the Thames and similar events were being organised on the Dee and the Trent

A further consequence of winter rowing was to question another of the accepted shibboleths, namely that there should be no rowing and certainly no racing on a Sunday. It was a point of view enshrined in the rules of university and college rowing on the Cam and a time-honoured convention on the Isis.[100] The ARA committee, most of whose members were brought up to honour the sabbath rule, was angry when the first Head of the River took place on a Sunday and informed its organisers that what they were doing was 'entirely contrary to the traditions and spirit of English amateur rowing.'[101] The delegates at the provincial meeting reacted even more strongly. The muscular Christians among them became very heated over the issue, one from Hereford RC declaring that 'the true spirit of amateur rowing and the true spirit of Christianity were so much alike that he should not wish to try to distinguish between them.'[102] Cynically, it might be noted that it was a convenient way of bolstering the middle-class image of the sport since those with little time for leisure would be unlikely to pursue an activity where the time available was so limited. Over the years the sabbath issue had led to discontent, argument and mutiny. Nottingham BC owed its foundation in 1894 to a secessionist group that objected to Nottingham RC's rigid insistence on preventing even pleasure boating on a Sunday.[103] At Derby RC, to break the rule was an offence that could lead to expulsion, while in 1927 Tyne ARC reinforced its strict view in the face of a revolt among some of its members.[104] A few clubs took a more liberal line. Evesham RC allowed its competitive crews to practice on a Sunday from 1912, while Wansbeck RC initially followed a similar line, allowing the boat-house to be open first until 12.30 p.m. and then until 4 p.m., until in 1925 the committee grew uneasy on the matter and withdrew the privilege.[105]

It would be easy to mock the stubborn committee members who insisted on guarding what some young Turks must have seen as rules deliberately designed to prevent progress. But many clubs owed their existence to the tolerant attitudes of the local community and it remained important still, especially during hard times, not to offend possibly sensitive susceptibilities. This was particularly the case over racing on Sundays. To have held a regatta on that day would have solved a great many difficulties. A constant problem facing the provincial meeting was the timetabling of races during a Saturday regatta. Until the Second World War it remained a common practice for offices and places of business to conduct their affairs on a Saturday morning and this could make nonsense of a regatta that started at ten or eleven in the morning.[106] To have held a regatta instead on a Sunday might have seemed a sensible alternative. But, leaving aside the point that to have levied a charge on the public would have meant a change in the law, such a move might have caused offence, in part to officials and competitors but above all, as one delegate at the 1927 provincial meeting put it, to 'the religious principles of a good many people which they had no right to do'. Whether he was right in his analysis is beside the point; he felt rowing could not take the risk. Another at the same meeting concluded 'that of all the public bodies governing sport, the Rowing Association should be the last and not the first to countenance racing on a Sunday'.[107] There is no evidence to suggest that the committee of the NARA would have disagreed with this conclusion.

V

English rowing then, during the first thirty or so years of this century, presented something of a tangled web. The fittest survived with some ease and considerable distinction. In the main these were the praetorian guard element within the ARA, less concerned than most by the besetting problems of the times. The years of depression emphasised that, in a good many cases, the foundations on which many of the smaller clubs were built were far from sound. The nature of the various tenancy agreements and the manifold difficulties of membership indicated that, at local level, the expansion at the end of the nineteenth century had not always been well conceived. Few of these less favoured clubs, not even the reasonably successful ones such as Derby and Agecroft, could contemplate the future with absolute certainty. For the rest, the constant periodic crises meant that by the 1920s their difficulties were being compounded. Paradoxically, because they had fewer pretensions and had not always committed themselves to the upkeep of capital equipment and buildings, many of the NARA clubs weathered the problems more easily than some of their ARA neighbours. The Falcon RC at Oxford, for example, enjoyed during the 1930s one of the more successful decades in its history.[108]

What, nevertheless, was remarkable about these difficult years was the number of clubs that did manage to survive. Fund-raising ventures, such as whist-drives and dances, may often have loomed larger than success at regattas but the kind of near-despair that afflicted Tees ABC in the mid-1920s and Stratford, a decade later, was unusual. There was a stubborn resilience that was impressive, a tribute to the devotion and the determination of club officials, however out of tune with the times and old-fashioned some of them may have seemed. In the course of it, a good many toes were no doubt trodden on but appearances were preserved and to the local community that could be important for the future. The Furnivall Scullers may have risked causing offence by rowing on Sundays but they continued to provide annual outings for some of the young and the old of Hammersmith, while the Tideway Boxing Day regatta always arranged for its surplus funds to be sent to a number of local hospitals. [109]

Whatever the divisions of opinions between the officials of the two associations, at the grass-roots level the reality was that most clubs, irrespective of their particular allegiance, had much in common with each other since they faced similar problems as well as the occasional taste of success and excitement. This was particular true of their rowing, whatever the standard they may have reached. G. O. Nickalls, son of a famous oarsman, holder of two Olympic silver medals and seven-times winner of the Grand at Henley, would have understood the simple pleasure of a former captain of St Philip's and St James's RC at Oxford who recalled the annual club races as 'the very jolliest hours of my life'. Such sentiments were not much different from Nickalls's own conclusion, that 'merely to glimpse these delights is something that makes rowing so very worthwhile'. [110] Given this kind of shared background, it was not totally surprising that advances began to be made towards healing divisions and that Nickalls was to play an important part in their final conclusion.

Notes

1 *The British Rowing Almanack*, 1923, pp. 170–1; Provincial Committee of the ARA *Minutes*, 17 September 1949. The spokesman was S. H. Johnson, a leading defender of the non-metropolitan clubs; C. S. Bell, *Derby Rowing Club – The First Hundred Years, 1879–1979* (Derby, 1979), p. 18.

2 NARA, *Minutes*, 23 November 1895.

3 *Ibid.*, 20 July 1895.

4 *Ibid.*, 26 November 1900.

5 *Ibid.*, 16 April 1904.

6 *Oxford Chronicle*, 10 August 1895.

7 Falcon R.C., *Minutes*, 19 February 1891.

8 NARA, *Minutes*, 1911, 'List of clubs'. The clubs were Trent RC at Burton, Nottingham Britannia, Broughton at Manchester, Jarrow RC, Mid-Tyne, also at Jarrow, Middlesbrough and York City.

9 *Ibid.*, 16 April 1904.
10 The relationship between the NARA and these regional associations can be gauged from the reports of *The Proceedings of the First, Second and Third Conferences of Amateur Rowing Associations, 1927, 1928* and *1929*. The West of England ARA was founded during 1895–6 following a suggestion that a Devon rowing association be formed. (See Exeter ARC, *Minutes*, 20 November 1895, 4 March 1896).
11 The TRCA is first mentioned in *The Almanack*, 1889, p. 182.
12 *The Almanack*, 1924, pp. 206, 208.
13 *Proceedings 1927*, pp. 11–2.
14 Tideway Boxing Day Charity Regatta, *Minutes*, 24 October 1929.
15 Weybridge RC, *Minutes*, 14 June 1924.
16 *Ibid.*, 19 May 1921.
17 NARA, *Report*, March 1924 – February 1925, p. 8.
18 *Proceedings 1927*, pp. 5–6.
19 NARA, *Minutes*, 9 April 1892.
20 *Proceedings 1928*, pp. 15–9, 66; *Proceedings 1929*, p. 18.
21 *Proceedings 1927*, pp. 15–9.
22 *Ibid.*, p. 5 and *Proceedings 1929*, p. 5.
23 *Proceedings 1929*, 'Summary of conclusions'.
24 Exeter ARC, *Minutes*, 7 March 1929.
25 The NARA from 1930 onwards consisted of the Hampshire and Dorset ARA, the Midland ARA, the North London ARA (the former Lea branch), the Norwich ARA, the Oxford ARA, the Thames ARA (the former Thames branch) and the West of England ARA. The coast ARA did not immediately join.
26 *The Almanack*, 1926, pp. 209–210; Tees ABC, *Minutes*, 5 April 1913, 8 June 1914, 7 April 1919, 5 June 1921; Middlesbrough ABC, *Minutes*, 30 December 1908. The problem was that the Durham committee appeared to have its own arbitrary rules governing the entry requirements for one event, the Corporation Challenge Cup. The failure to clear this matter up according to ARA rules meant that the two Tees clubs boycotted Durham Regatta for a number of years.
27 *The Almanack*, 1927, p. 198.
28 *Ibid.*, 1929, pp. 173–4. The immediate cause of the outburst was the apparent failure of the ARA to indicate to Nottingham and Union the rules about the weight of coxes at the 1928 Olympic Regatta where the Nottingham crew had represented Great Britain. The ARA at this time had little interest in coxed four rowing.
29 Provincial Committee of the ARA, *Minutes* 2 December 1933.
30 NARA *Annual Report 1931*, passim.
31 J. A. King, *compiler, A Short History of Kingston Rowing Club, 1858–1983* (London, 1983), pp. 13–4.
32 London RC, *Reports*, 1924–35, p. 92.
33 *Ibid.*, 1871, *passim*; Thames RC, *Minutes*, 13 March 1875.
34 K. Tarbuck, ed., *Liverpool Victoria 1884–1934 – Jubilee Souvenir* (privately printed, 1934), pp. 11–2.
35 *Ibid.*, p. 17.

36 Weybridge RC, *Minutes*, 25 January, 5 February, 26 March 1922.
37 Middlesbrough ABC, *Minutes*, 2 July, 2 October, 1 November, 11 December 1900, 15 February, 28 March, 15 April, 4 June 1901.
38 *Exeter Express and Echo*, 15 April 1964.
39 R. J. Davis, *Boating at Worcester in the Nineteenth Century* (Worcester, undated), p. 36.
40 Neil Wigglesworth, *Rowing in the North West* (unpublished M.Ed. thesis, Manchester University 1983), pp. 75–6.
41 Anonymous, *Walton RC* (privately printed, 1977), p. 14; Tees ABC, *Minutes*, 15 April, 6 June 1932, May 1946.
42 Exeter A.R.C., *Minutes*, 6 May 1946.
43 *Stratford-upon-Avon Herald*, 12 March 1937.
44 Stratford-upon-Avon BC, *Minutes*, 12 June 1882, 8 June 1885.
45 Durham ARC, Minutes, 7 March 1891; Middlesbrough ABC, *Minutes*, 8, 17 October 1895, 10 February 1898.
46 Exeter ARC, *Minutes*, 6 April 1905; Weybridge RC, Minutes, 20 April 1921, 23 April 1922.
47 Evesham RC, Minutes, 26 September 1930, 20 March 1931, 16 March, 19 June 1934.
48 *Stratford-upon-Avon Herald*, 12 March 1937, reporting the AGM of Stratford BC on 8 March 1937.
49 Stratford-upon-Avon BC, *Minutes*, 2 March 1934, 23 April 1935, 8 March 1937.
50 Exeter ARC, *Minutes*, 28 September, 26 October 1928.
51 Wansbeck RC, *Minutes*, 1 June 1911, 2 June 1912.
52 C. M. Ainslie, *A History of the Falcon Rowing Clubs* (typescript, Oxford City Libraries, 1969), p. 3.
53 Tees ABC, *Minutes*, 3 May 1920, 22 March 1926.
54 C. S. Bell, *Derby Rowing Club – The First Hundred Years 1879–1979* (Derby, 1979), pp. 17–8.
55 Tyne ARC, *Minutes*, 27 November 1928.
56 J. Gretton, *et al.*, *Derwent Rowing Club – Centenary 1857–1957* (Derby, 1957), p. 8; Bell, *Derby Rowing Club*, p. 59.
57 Tarbuck, *Liverpool Victoria*, p. 21.
58 Tyne ARC *Minutes*, 20 March 1936; Evesham RC *Minutes*, 15 July 1932, 6 April 1933, 12 April 1935.
59 Wigglesworth, *Rowing in the North West*, pp. 76–7.
60 Exeter ARC, *Minutes*, 26 September 1929.
61 *The Almanack*, 1906, pp. 196–7.
62 Durham ARC, *Minutes*, 19 December 1913.
63 Gretton, *Derwent Rowing Club*, p. 6.
64 *John Johnson Collection*, Bodleian Library, Box 13, Wargrave Regatta cards for August 1898 and August 1901; Evesham RC, *Minutes*, 23 March, 16 April 1909.
65 H. Cleaver, *A History of Rowing* (London, 1957), pp. 156–9.
66 Furnivall Sculling Club, *Minutes*, 25 March 1925.
67 Dora Falconer, *Women's University Rowing between World Wars I and II* (undated typescript), *passim*.

68 Exeter ARC, *Minutes*, 5 July 1950.
69 Tees ABC, *Minutes*, 23 January 1925.
70 *Ibid.*, April (no day recorded), 1925.
71 Middlesbrough A.B.C., *Cash Account, 1901–2*, 24 March 1902.
72 Durham ARC, *Letter Book*, 11 December 1902; Evesham RC, *Minutes*, 10 August 1909; Furnivall Sculling Club, *Minutes*, 14 May 1913.
73 Nottingham RC, *Minutes*, 6 September 1899.
74 Tyne ARC, *Minutes*, 11 July 1910.
75 Evesham RC, *Minutes*, 18 July 1920, 19 February 1932, 30 May 1938.
76 Stratford-upon-Avon BC, *Minutes*, 22 April 1935.
77 *The Almanack*, 1927, p. 192.
78 Beresford won gold medals in the 1924 Olympic sculls, the 1932 coxswainless fours and the 1936 double sculls. He won a silver in the 1920 single sculls and in the 1928 eights final. In addition, he won ten Henley medals, including four in the Diamonds, held the Wingfield Sculls on seven occasions and in 1924 and 1925 the Philadelphia Gold Cup, at that time the amateur championship of the world.
79 R. D. Burnell, *Swing Together – Thoughts on Rowing* (London, 1952), Chapter 2, *passim*.
80 Eighth AGM of the Provincial Rowing Clubs, 1928, pp. 4–5.
81 NARA, *Handbook for 1937*, p. 6. The losing sculler was W. E. C. Horwood of Chiswick Generals RC, his opponent being H. L. Warren of Trinity Hall, Cambridge.
82 *Newcastle Journal*, 20 May 1939.
83 Bell, *Derby Rowing Club*, pp. 12, 18–23.
84 W. A. Locan, *The Agecroft Story, 1861–1960* (Salford, 1960), pp. 36–8, 40–5.
85 During 1927–35, for example, London RC rowed twice in Paris, once in Denmark, Belgium and Portugal and in 1934 in Australia. London RC, *Reports, 1924–1935, passim*.
86 *The Almanack*, 1907, pp. 227–8.
87 *Ibid.*, 1911, pp. 198–9.
88 Sixth AGM of the Provincial Rowing Clubs, 1926, p. 13.
89 Eighth AGM of the Provincial Rowing Clubs, 1928, pp. 6–7.
90 *Ibid.*, p. 7.
91 *Ibid.*, 1926, p. 13.
92 See, for example, Fairbairn's letter to *The Times* of 9 June 1927 after he had been accused of only producing men capable of rowing fast over a short distance but worthless for something like the Boat Race. 'This is quite wrong.' he wrote, 'Since I began coaching Jesus, Cambridge in 1905, that college has got more blues than any other except Trinity; and leaving out Trinity, Trinity Hall, St. John's and Pembroke, Jesus has got more blues than all the sixteen other colleges put together – that is sixteen colleges, orthodoxly coached, cannot get as many blues as one college coached by me, or my style is fully sixteen times as good as the orthodox style for getting blues.'
93 Tideway Boxing Day Charity Regatta, *Minutes*, 30 August, 13 November 1922, 9 November 1925, 24 October 1929, 24 April 1930.
94 Weybridge RC, *Minutes*, 30 September 1923.
95 Furnivall Sculling Club, *Minutes*, 8 January 1932.

96 Nottingham RC, *Minutes*, 8 September 1909; Tees ABC, *Minutes*, 25 February 1921.
97 *The Almanack*, 1924, p. 18.
98 *Ibid.*, 1927, p. 17; London RC, *Reports, 1924–35*, pp. 4–5.
99 London RC, *Reports, 1924–35*, p. 46.
100 R. C. Lehmann, *The Complete Oarsman*, (London, 1908), Appendix IV – 'Rules and regulations of CUBC'.
101 *The Almanack*, 1928, pp. 190–1.
102 Seventh AGM of the Provincial Rowing Clubs, 1927, pp. 5–7.
103 R. A. Church, *Economic and Social Change in a Midland Town; Victorian Nottingham, 1815–1900* (London, 1966), pp. 376–7.
104 Bell, *Derby Rowing Club*, p. 3; Tyne ARC, *Minutes*, 3 March 1927.
105 Evesham RC, *Minutes*, 14 May 1912; Wansbeck RC, *Minutes*, June 1911, 6 August 1925.
106 Eighth AGM of the Provincial Rowing Clubs, 1928, pp. 8–9 and tenth AGM, 1930, pp. 7–9.
107 Seventh AGM of the Provincial Rowing Clubs, 1927, pp. 5–6.
108 Ainslie, *Falcon Rowing Clubs*, p. 2.
109 Furnivall Scullers Appeal, 11 May 1896 in *John Johnson Collection*, Box 13; Furnivall Sculling Club, *Minutes*, 24 March 1912; Tideway Boxing Day Charity Regatta, *Minutes*, 8 October 1924.
110 Anonymous, *The Record of the Rowing Club of St Philip and St James, Oxford, 1889–1909* (Oxford, 1910), p. 17; G. O. Nickalls, *A Rainbow in the Sky – Reminiscences* (London, 1974), p. 148.

7

Fusion and unity

Speaking at the 1927 NARA conference, its chairman, Prebendary Propert, expressed the hope that the ARA would eventually recognise the validity of 'our definition and come into line. I have spoken to many men who belong to A.R.A. clubs and they are in sympathy and agreement with us.'[1] Given that many clubs, whatever their allegiance, shared common problems and difficulties, the probability is that Propert was correct, but, unfortunately, there were no signs during the 1920s that the main ARA committee was likely to seek an accommodation on the amateur issue. Contact between the two associations was kept to a minimum and what there was, as over the Peace Regatta in 1919 and the 1920 Olympics, was bitter and acrimonious. There seemed little hope of reconciliation. That degree of tolerance that had followed R. C. Lehmann's initiative in 1894 seemed by the 1920s to have been eroded and the ARA, in the shape of its committee, stood magisterially aloof. It looked as if the hidebound element within the praetorian guard had at last gained the ascendancy. There was to be no tampering with the definition of an amateur and there appeared little prospect of ending the dual form of government.

Yet, within ten years of Propert's pious statement, the two associations were talking to each other and the manual labour clause was about to be removed from the ARA definition. This change of heart admits of no simple explanation. Shifts in social attitudes during the 1930s, following the worst effects of the depression, might seem to provide the essential clue. But in the end, the solution has to be found amongst those in the seat of power, in this case the more rigid members of the ARA committee.

I

The depression had brought uneven consequences. In many cases it had simply underlined the basic fragility of many of the clubs, a weakness already obvious among some of them before 1914. For the majority there had certainly been a degree of shared misery that had served to minimise differences. But the effects of this are easy to exaggerate since in many parts of the country members of the two associations rarely came across each other. In the West Country, for example, the NARA through the West of England ARA had a virtual monopoly, while elsewhere, as in the North East, it had no influence whatsoever by 1920. Nor ought the authority of either of the associations to be exaggerated, more particularly when it came to providing solutions to some of the difficulties of the inter-war period. The discussions of the main ARA committee, for example, are empty of reference to the kinds of problems facing a good many of its constituent clubs. It had in any case little of substance to offer. Neither of the associations had complete control over its member clubs, the realisation of which was largely responsible for prompting the NARA to consider reorganisation in 1930. Even so, more effective as its structure became, it lacked resources to assist those in difficulty and depended ultimately on the goodwill and co-operation of the local associations and clubs.

The ARA on the other hand never contemplated any kind of reorganisation since there seemed no pressing need for reform. It continued to grow slowly but its power-base remained the metropolitan Thames, the Isis and the Cam. In 1923 Derby RC, one of the more successful and soundly based of the provincial clubs, decided to affiliate to the ARA and it seems to have been a calculated gesture to increase its influence locally.[2] That Derby can have expected anything more seems unlikely but in any case the ARA had little to offer other than membership of an association that granted a cachet of respectability. Yet there were a number of warning signs of dissatisfaction, specifically over the issue of the amateur definition. Reading Regatta had an inconsistent and fitful record, disappearing only to be revived again on a number of occasions. By the early 1920s it was once again in difficulties and in 1922 its committee recorded that the only solution to low numbers entering for the regatta was to persuade the ARA to be less rigid.[3] To those involved in organising the affair, it seemed self-evident that the sinking of differences was the only way to revive the sport at provincial level. Others were of the same opinion. In June 1923 the ARA committee expressed its alarm that officials at the regattas held at Evesham, Stratford and Burton were admitting crews from unaffiliated clubs without sufficient scrutiny of the oarsmen's credentials.[4] The implications that those regattas were allowing entries that did not fulfil the strict ARA definition was obvious. But the Midlands area had a long tradition, dating back to the early 1880s, of irritating the ARA and of ignoring when it saw fit its more cherished precepts. But, at a time when a significant number of unaffiliated clubs existed or where there was an alternative organisation, the ARA had few powers to enforce its rulings. This was underlined in March 1933 by its reaction to a letter from the Northern Rowing Council, representative of north-eastern clubs of which none, apart from one, belonged to either association. The ARA was told 'that in the opinion of this council, members of the constabulary are eligible to row as amateurs in regattas held under the jurisdiction of the N.A.R.C.'. The reply indicated how feeble was the ARA's real authority. It simply acknowledged the letter as an expression of opinion, pointing out that it was contrary to all previous rulings.[5] In fact there was absolutely nothing in the circumstances that the ARA could do to enforce its own decisions if the authorities in a particular area decided to disregard them. It was but one further indication that at grass-roots level, clubs and regattas were prepared to ignore rules and regulations that seemed calculated to impede rather than to encourage the sport.

Whenever the occasion allowed, there was some degree of help and co-operation between clubs of the two associations that in no way broke any of the codes of practice. Weybridge RC, for example, in addition to having Steve Fairbairn as one of the coaches of its 1924 Olympic four, borrowed equipment from ARA clubs. Vesta RC lent an eight for the Desborough Cup in 1925, while Merton College seems to have helped Weybridge oarsmen whenever they visited Oxford Royal Regatta.[6] Opportunities for this kind of collaboration were most obvious on the Thames and it was there that the most fruitful areas of co-operation developed during the 1920s and 1930s. The nature of the Tideway Boxing Day Charity Regatta meant that crews from the ARA, the NARA, the Tradesmen's RCA and later, the Women's ARA, all participated. Each had its own separate event but representatives of the different codes all met on its committee. Throughout the 1920s the chairman was an ARA man, H. T. Blackstaffe of Vesta RC, winner of the Wingfields and the Diamonds and holder of a gold medal from the 1908 Olympic Regatta. Charles Tugwell was one of the NARA members, while W. H. Eyre, the well-known Thames RC oarsman of the previous century, was one of the vice-presidents.[7] Harmony and understanding, apart from some initial hesitation about the presence of women, were the characteristics of this unique regatta. It was a fruitful and important experiment.

It must be a matter of surmise as to just how important mutual self-help and co-operation of this kind actually was. No doubt the more obstinate members of the ARA committee were unlikely to take very much notice of tow-path decision-makers. But they ought at least to have reflected on their possible worth given the open sympathy for some revision of the amateur definition by a formidable trio of old oarsmen. One was Lord Iveagh, a winner of the Wingfields, who became patron of the NARA, and another was R.C. Bourne, one of the most successful of Oxford strokes, MP for that city, and a consistent supporter of the local regatta as well as an NARA vice-president. The third and most well-known was Lord Desborough, formerly W. H. Grenfell, Oxford blue and Henley steward. He may have been opposed to the presence of foreign crews at Henley but he remained unhappy about the manner in which the ARA treated the NARA, making his point by presenting the latter with its most important championship trophy.[8] Such magnanimity was a forceful reminder to some of those on the ARA committee that there was a larger vision than that contained by the banks of the Isis, the Cam and the Tideway.

II

The change when it came was almost unexpected, although in 1935 there had been an important sign of some softening of attitude on the part of the praetorian guard. In that year – and the practice continued until 1939 – the Henley stewards agreed to leave the booms along the regatta course to allow the NARA to hold its annual championships. It was a small but welcome gesture and was greatly appreciated by the NARA.[9] Such generosity, however, seemed to be denied the next year by the refusal of the Australian eight's entry for the Grand Challenge Cup on the grounds that they were policemen and therefore ineligible. The Henley stewards in fact had no choice in the matter. They had to obey their own rules and there was no way in which they could immediately disentangle themselves from a web of their own making. It was an embarrassing incident since British oarsmen, all of them from the ARA camp, would be likely to race the Australians a few weeks later at the Olympic Regatta at Berlin. Nor was the situation improved when questions were raised about the issue in Parliament.[10] The ARA in its turn, whatever its crabbed views about Olympic competition, can hardly have found much consolation in the performance of its crews at Berlin. It called into question the wisdom of basing international selection on such a narrow band of oarsmen.[11] Had the ARA and Henley authorities had any knowledge of their own history, they might have recalled that their original definition of an amateur had been much influenced by the need to accommodate overseas crews competing in this country. Once again, the foreign issue was to play a decisive part in forcing further modification.

Two elements therefore were coinciding. The first was the realisation by the ARA that among the clubs and individual oarsmen, there was unease at the continued insistence on the rigidity of the amateur rule. It was, in fact, once more becoming an object of some public debate. The president of Southampton University College BC wrote to *The Times* explaining that a generous patron had presented a cup for competition by all clubs on the River Itchen. But, if the Southampton students took part, they were liable to be disqualified and barred since their opponents belonged in the main to the NARA. He concluded by suggesting that 'the time has come for real brotherhood in what is to many of us the finest sport for young men'.[12] W. H. Eyre, recalling his days on the main ARA committee, deplored the tangled and perverse arguments often used to debar someone from joining an ARA club, while the Reverend Sidney Swann, former Cambridge blue and for long involved with the NARA, pointed to foreign successes at Henley and for the need to exploit 'the very best that England can produce, whether they happen to work with their heads or with their hands'.[13]

Swann's emphasis on the strength of overseas crews, coming as it did after the disappointments at Berlin, touched a raw nerve but reminded people of the other element in the equation. The ARA, once so confident, was suddenly vulnerable as the divine right of its best crews to defend successfully the country's reputation was questioned. Charles Tugwell, as secretary of the NARA, timed his approach with some skill. At its meeting in April 1936, the full council of the NARA had agreed that an approach to the ARA over the amateur issue was worth contemplating. There must have been some doubt and hesitation at that particular time as to whether the ARA would respond sympathetically, but, by delaying until November, Tugwell was able to take advantage of the general alarm in its ranks over the events of the summer. The ARA promptly agreed to a conference in February 1937 and both sides appointed their representatives.[14]

As had happened at the meeting forty-six years earlier, the NARA side, this time in the person of Tugwell, took the initiative. The difference was that the ARA members were in a far less sanguine mood than on the first occasion. Tugwell, after flattering the ARA as 'the most influential rowing body in the world', reminded the meeting of the position during the early 1890s. He claimed – and by and large he was right – that nobody had really disputed the validity of the ARA definition at that time and that all the NARA had wanted was some form of recognition. Tugwell, by refreshing the ARA's memory in this way, was drawing attention to the degree of tolerance that had once existed between the two associations and which had apparently been lost during the years following the Great War. He then reminded the meeting of the manner in which the ARA had over the years drawn the line of acceptability far lower on the social scale than might have been expected: 'With the passage of time, you have not altered the letter of your rules, but you have altered the spirit of them by accepting such men as sorters, telegraphists, shop assistants, clerks etc.' The conclusion, he argued, was obvious. At a time when Parliament was actively pursuing legislation to improve the physical fitness of the nation and when the Duke of York's camp at Romney Marsh was bringing together young men and boys from widely different social backgrounds, it was surely time to modify the rules. He concluded:

> that an organisation such as the Amateur Rowing Association, with which so many people of influence are connected, should, in this Coronation year, feel that it was incumbent upon them to support the efforts of Royalty and to make a gesture of goodwill by placing the definition of an amateur oarsman upon a sound and universally accepted basis – a basis whereby any man who rows for the love of the sport, and does not get any advantage by his employment in or about boats, or is not a professional, should be able to row under one definition, an amateur definition that would be acceptable to all concerned and give offence to none, and one that would sweep away any suggestion of class prejudice.

It was a shrewd and calculated piece, not delving into private grief by reminding the ARA of its international inadequacies but instead appealing to its members' conscience and underlining that both associations believed in the virtues of the amateur ideal and basically accepted the same rules. At the end of it, C. M. Pitman, the ARA chairman, admitted that he could no longer defend his association's view on an amateur. The agreement was, therefore, made to remove the manual labour clause and to allow crews to row in each other's events.[15]

The meeting had been hedged about with some secrecy. The NARA representatives had the support of their AGM from the previous year but the ARA claimed that they needed further time, especially to consult the stewards at Henley. The ARA had no intention of widening the debate any further since, it claimed, its committee was fully representative and there was, as a result, no need to consult the clubs further or to hold a referendum.[16] On 9 June, the ARA committee drew up its recommendations and they were accepted the following day by the stewards at Henley, meeting under Lord Desborough's chairmanship. On 11 June an announcement was made setting out the new ARA definition of an amateur and the consequent changes of rules as well as the fact that Henley had also consented to them. At the same time the NARA agreed to the changes so that, for the first time, irrespective of the association to which they belonged, all oarsmen could compete in each other's regattas, including Henley.[17] The two bodies had moved very close to each other but there was at the time no hint of fusion, both preserving their separate organisations and identities. *The Times*, welcomed the end of 'this anachronism, reminiscent of obsolete social distinctions' and optimistically drew the conclusion that nobody had dared to mention at the joint meeting, that 'there is every prospect of increasing cooperation between the two associations, to the benefit of both and of English rowing as a whole'.[18]

III

Such immediate hopes were not to be realised, in part because of the outbreak of war in 1939. But, in any case, the different programmes of the two associations did not easily allow for much greater co-operation than already existed. A NARA eight from the Metropolitan Police entered for the Thames Cup at Henley in 1938 and an ARA club, Henley RC, won the open eights at the NARA championship.[19] But the main point about the 1937 negotiations and agreement had been the ending of a grievance as far as the NARA was concerned and the removal of a source of embarrassment to the ARA. For most of the clubs, the effects seem to have been minimal.

The settling of the main issue between the two bodies seems equally to have left them both uncertain about what should be their future attitudes to each other. There was a general feeling that contact at official level should be maintained but it was not at all clear what matters should be discussed. A Joint Co-ordinating Committee was set up and met in

February 1939 arriving at conclusions that were limp at best. There was some talk about the design of rowing tanks and what was the effective life for various kinds of boats and oars. On only one issue was there firm agreement and that had nothing to do at all with rowing, namely their united condemnation of the views of the Oxford Group Movement, later known as Moral Rearmament.[20] A good deal more important was the ARA's decision in the spring of 1939 to approach both the NARA and the Scottish Rowing Association with the idea of setting up a British Rowing Board that could become affiliated to FISA.[21] The onset of war prevented the idea being pursued any further but it was a measure of the changing attitudes within the ARA that it should have been suggested at all.

From the perspective of the clubs the most significant development was the passing in 1937 of the Physical Training and Recreation Act. Its aim was to provide the means for a fuller and fitter life for people of all ages and to improve facilities for sport and recreation throughout England and Wales. A National Advisory Council under Lord Aberdare was appointed to advise the government on these matters as well as a Grants Committee to recommend to the Board of Education, responsible for administering the Act, what kind of financial help should be given. Within the terms of the Act, a grant was provided enabling Charles Tugwell to be appointed as National Organiser for Rowing. The original appointment was for twelve months only, although it was in fact renewed, and the ARA committee raised no objection either to the title or to the man appointed. Indeed, once Tugwell had made it clear that he did not mean to confine his activities to the NARA clubs, the ARA agreed to contribute to his expenses.[22] The anonymous editor of *The Almanack* spoke of the solution to the amateur issue and Tugwell's appointment under the Physical Training Scheme in one and the same breath. Together they appeared to mark for the first time some degree of common purpose among all amateur oarsmen in the country.[23]

A large number of clubs responded to this government-sponsored initiative though not all were able to take advantage of its terms. Some of the NARA clubs discovered that there was no proper safeguards in their constitutions guaranteeing that their boat-houses would continue to be used for rowing in the foreseeable future. A solution was quickly found by having the NARA incorporated under the Companies Act of 1929 so that club boat-houses could be vested in the new company which would act as the legal trustee.[24] It was an ingenious arrangement that in the end guaranteed Weybridge RC a small grant after it became entangled in bureaucratic buck-passing between the scheme's administrators and the local council over the conditions of its short-term lease.[25] None of the clubs on the Tees were granted any money but they received a sympathetic hearing from Tugwell who urged them to reconsider amalgamation as a way out of their individual difficulties. He saw enough to be impressed by their enthusiasm and arranged for Ernest Barry, the professional oarsman, to spend most of June 1939 on the Tees coaching and training the crews.[26] Given its relatively sound base, it might seem unjust that Evesham RC obtained a grant while those on the Tees were refused one.[27] But it was part of Tugwell's unenviable lot to encourage success and not to waste public money on ventures that might prove vulnerable. As it was, ninety-six clubs and associations submitted plans, the total cost of which would have been just over £111,000. Not all of them were accepted and others were withdrawn because of the terms governing the grants but Tugwell was able to recommend the disbursement of over £21,500.[28] It was by no means a large sum but, had the war not intervened, the probability is that the assistance would have been greater in future years.

An unforeseen consequence of Tugwell's appointment was that he became the best informed official, in either association, about the real state of affairs among the smaller and, in particular, the provincial clubs. This gave him considerable authority and, during his travels throughout the country, he began to assume the role of a benevolent consultant to those with serious problems. One particular group especially attracted his attention, those residual professional oarsmen who still existed on parts of the Thames and in the North East. He was already well informed about the former and had contacts with the Tradesmen's RCA through the committee of the Boxing Day Regatta. He retained considerable respect for the expertise of many of them, such as Ernest Barry, but was quick to see that, given the potential growth of amateur rowing following the agreement between the ARA and the NARA, they were out of the mainstream of events. In the North East, however, he found the professionals there already virtually isolated. Their standard was poor, their equipment was old and their morale low. Arguments abounded as witness the meeting in October 1938 to discuss the future of the Christmas Sculling Handicap where, according to one who was present, 'the apparent uneasy atmosphere present had such an effect that no chairman was appointed.'[29]

Tugwell attended a meeting at Newcastle in November 1938 to discuss with the local professional clubs how they could benefit from the National Fitness Scheme. His immediate advice was to encourage them to form their own organisation to safeguard their own particular interests and to provide an opportunity for the discussion of matters of common concern.[30] It quickly became obvious that the one issue he wanted them to consider was whether there was any point in their remaining professionals at all. The first meeting of what became known as the Northern Rowing Association was held in April 1939 and the former Oxford blue, G. J. P. Merifield, was asked to take the chair. The main purpose was to consider and accept a constitution for the association which Tugwell had taken the trouble to prepare. It offered the oarsmen an ingenious way out of their dilemma, one which gave some hope that in the fullness of time they could be accepted as amateurs by the NARA. His scheme began with the premise that the only oarsmen who would be debarred from the new NRA would be those who had rowed 'for personal profit'.[31] It was obvious that few of them could claim to have done that, especially if expenses were deducted from the meagre winnings. In some cases clubs had not won a money prize within living memory and, in Merifield's judgement, could hardly be called professional at all.[32] The basic principle, stated bluntly by Merifield as being 'to get the northern professional clubs onto an amateur status', was accepted by all those present at the meeting, though the discussion was long and arduous since they were being asked to abandon a proud and ancient heritage.[33] But the good sense of the move was recognised and to the treasurer of the new organisation, Jack Briggs, gave renewed hope for the future. So excited was he at these prospects that he took his sculling boat down to the Newcastle quayside and, veteran though he may have been, attracted the attention of the crowd that was always there on a Sunday morning by a series of acrobatics and then urged any young man among them to join a rowing club.[34]

Charles Tugwell interpreted his brief as National Organiser for Rowing as widely as he dared and in this he was right. Nobody before had been given the opportunity of judging the state of all rowing in the country and, in the particular case of the north-eastern professionals, he saw a group which could easily become its outcasts. It was something that he was determined to avoid. His vision was a wide one but he was sufficiently shrewd to realise that in a matter of this nature he must move with caution. To have suggested in 1939 that such clubs as the Empire RC at Gateshead and Cambois RC, as the Wansbeck club now called itself, could be mentioned in the same breath as Leander and London RC would have seemed outrageous. But that one day they could all row against each other remained for Tugwell a real possibility, one that he was prepared to work towards carefully and tenaciously.

IV

Inevitably the Second World War delayed the promise of the 1937 agreement. On the face of it, the circumstances that greeted peace again in 1945 ought to have hastened the fulfilment of greater accord between the ARA and the NARA. A reforming government came into power and there seemed little likelihood of that rapid withering away of hopes and expectations that had marked the aftermath of the Great War. In spite of shortages and a continuation of rationing, the desire for a 'New Jerusalem' that would reflect the nation's sacrifices was not to be gainsaid. The fact that the country could hardly afford it was ignored.

It is hard to find much evidence of similar idealism in the rowing world in the immediate post-war years. Pragmatism, poverty as well as some confidence, mingled together a little uncertainly. A good many clubs had closed down or had drastically curtailed their activities during the war but in a few places some rowing had continued. The outbreak of war in 1914 had led many oarsmen to volunteer immediately but the more measured pattern of conscription from 1939 onwards allowed some degree of continuity. Agecroft RC actually benefited when ICI research workers, a few with university experience, joined the club and allowed some competitive rowing to continue throughout the war years.[35] The same was true at Evesham where the membership had increased to such proportions by 1945 that there was talk of imposing a limit.[36] Weybridge RC perspicaciously began to recruit young members with a view to the future.[37] Such resilience led immediately after 1945 to a renewal of full activities and reflected the sound base that had been established by many such clubs during the inter-war period.

The effects of direct enemy action, however, could test the resources of any club. The boat-house of the Empire RC was hit by a bomb on the night of 5 May 1941 and everything was destroyed.[38] During one night of October 1940, the elegant boat-house of the Furnivall Scullers on the Mall at Hammersmith was badly damaged by a bomb and the problem was exacerbated by looters. In July 1943, the empty building was further shaken by a flying bomb that fell nearby. Without the friendly assistance of the National Provincial Bank RC and the Linden RC, the club would probably have collapsed.[39] The destruction of the Empire RC premises was enough to persuade the Tyne ARC to sell most of its boats during 1942 since there seemed no guarantee of their security.[40] Such action reflected that air of uncertainty that had affected the club for most of the inter-war years. It made recovery after 1945 all the more difficult. The same was true on the River Tees. There the Tees ABC boat-house had collapsed not through enemy action but because of bad weather and neglect. It turned members' attention once more to the possibility of fusion with the equally miserable Middlesbrough club and in 1946 this was at last agreed as being the best hope for the future.[41] The same solution was considered on the Exe and in the same year Port Royal ARC and Exeter RC joined together.[42] A similar proposal was mooted among the various city clubs at Oxford, if only on a temporary basis to meet immediate local needs. In the end, the scheme was developed along different lines as a limited company to plan for a communal boat-house for all the clubs.[43]

For some, the return to normality after the war seemed smooth and effortless. At the Olympic Regatta held at Henley in 1948, British crews won two gold and a silver medal, suggesting that the praetorian guard was quickly re-finding its form. Provincial coxed fours – from Agecroft, Evesham, Newark, Royal Chester, Stourport and Stratford – rowed together in an Olympic trial and, although none was selected, their standard suggested that in the Midlands area there was considerable and commendable vigour.[44] Others, whether through mischance or misjudgement, found recovery a good deal more difficult. The Furnivall Scullers had spent the grant given to them in 1942 by the War Damage Commission on settling a number of outstanding debts. They had little money left to play with, found it hard to find good second-hand equipment and were restricted in their membership as long as they were the guests of another club. In addition, they found themselves faced by differing planning demands as they contemplated the task of rebuilding their damage boat-house.[45] The meeting of the Empire RC in October 1946 was succinct in the way it reported its problems. The club needed a new site, a new boat-house, boats and oars. Some £750 was available from the government because of bomb damage and interest would be paid as from 1941 as long as the club did not seek advance payments.[46] In an attempt to revive the activities of the small clubs along the river, Tyne United RC was set up in February 1946 to provide the remaining members of the Empire, Hawthorn, Gateshead and District and Walker and Wallsend clubs with some rowing. In the circumstances, the new club, intended only to be temporary, was seen as the only possible permanent solution available.[47] Tyne ARC found its boat-house in better shape than had been expected but had little money available for any kind of equipment. Nevertheless, with praiseworthy stoicism, it decided to hold its annual regatta in 1947.[48] The new Tees club was without a site for a boat-house and, like others, in need of new resources of almost every description. It found itself, for example, with much that was incompatible – oars made for fixed rowlocks and boats with swivel pins. There was indignation when it was discovered that Chester-le-Street RC, an old professional club, had received a grant from the recently formed Central Council for Physical Recreation while the Tees club did not qualify because it had so little to show for itself. It decided to seek the advice of the NARA as to the way forward but, in fact, its problems and dilemmas were to be solved only by its own hard work and a great deal of faith.[49] In essence, clubs such as the Furnivall Scullers, Tees and Tyne United, and to some extent also Tyne ARC, were new creations. Assuming they could rid themselves of old prejudices, there were some advantages in having what was virtually a clean slate.

Those associated with the ARA found little guidance from the main committee which had never concerned itself with the business of running a club or a regatta except when a serious breach of the rules was brought to its notice. Some degree of tension certainly existed since it appeared to some that the ARA, along with the stewards at Henley, remained still largely interested in the activities of the elite clubs. One issue in particular served to channel what was mainly provincial resentment. Until 1873 all fours events at Henley and elsewhere had been in coxed boats but, after the advent of the coxswainless variety, the older type was relegated, at least as far as the elite clubs were concerned, to second-class status. But in the great majority of clubs, the coxed four remained the chosen type of boat and the only one suitable for most English rivers and regattas with their narrow and twisting courses. After 1945, considerable pressure was exerted by the representatives of the provincial clubs on the ARA in the hope that Henley might be persuaded to institute an event for such boats. The argument was clear enough. Such a competition, it was felt, would encourage and raise the standard of rowing throughout the country and might enable some of the less well-known to seek international representation.[50] The consistent refusal of the stewards to entertain the idea and the lukewarm attitude of the ARA in pressing the matter caused considerable resentment. All that the latter managed to do was to introduce during the 1950s a coxed four championship that was hawked round various regattas without ever being very successful. If anything, it increased the degree of indignation. At the 1952 meeting of the provincial ARA clubs, a serious attempt was made to make the annual levy on all oarsmen towards the cost of international competition conditional on the provision of a coxed four event at Henley. G. O. Nickalls, the chairman of the ARA who was present, had to use all his skills to quash this incipient rebellion, reminding the meeting that the ARA was not responsible for what went on at Henley Royal Regatta.[51]

Discontent of this kind was real enough. It was not always well articulated and consisted in the main of half-truths and tow-path grousing. Those expressing themselves in this way ignored two points. The first was the one that Nickalls had already made, namely that it was not the practice of the ARA to interfere with how a particular regatta was run. The second was more complex, concerned with the internal workings of the main ARA committee itself. It was a peculiarly unrepresentative body, largely as the result of history. Nine clubs, with some 5,500 members, had seventeen delegates. These were the so-called nominating clubs, those most concerned with the setting up of the ARA during the early 1880s. Another seventy clubs, largely the smaller ones along the Thames, Lea and the Medway, with some 5,000 members, nominated three representatives, while the remaining seventy-two clubs in the provinces, with a membership of about 6,000, had a further six places on the committee.[52] If the bulk of the membership had cause for genuine complaint, it might have been here. Yet, in 1937, nobody had objected when the ARA had changed the amateur rule without any form of consultation other than with the Henley stewards. Nevertheless, the volunteer officers of the association – by the early 1950s, Nickalls as chairman and J. H. Page as secretary – were forced to manoeuvre with skill and sensitivity because of the preponderance on the committee of the elite club representatives. These men had moved a long way in 1937 and for some of them it had been the equivalent of coming off the gold standard. That major point of principle, the heart of the message advanced by Selwyn, Shadwell and Egan, one which had for so long shaped and governed attitudes and practices, had suddenly disappeared. The temptation, therefore, for the ARA officers to run for cover behind the praetorian guard was a real one, all the more so when the elite clubs in the immediate aftermath of the war appeared once again to have re-established their effortless superiority. That the ARA did not lapse once more into becoming the mouthpiece of a small group of clubs was, in large measure, the result of the way that Nickalls and Page handled the main committee. Criticism of the kind made over the coxed four issue may have reflected the genuine worries of the many that the few might covertly opt for a conservative stance. But they did not make the task of Nickalls and Page any easier as they tried to balance the conflicting demands of the various groups that now made up the ARA.

V

The NARA, in the person of its secretary Charles Tugwell, must have been well aware of some of the strains and tensions within the main ARA committee and of the dangers likely to arise if he were to move too quickly. Writing in the 1948 *Almanack*, he went no further than to point out the outstanding differences between the two associations and to express the hope that in the not too distant future there might be some form of co-ordinating body for all domestic rowing.[53] His own personal accord with the ARA officials was a good one but he was more aware than most that, at a grass-roots level, the 1937 agreement had, as yet, had little effect with clubs from the two associations still pursuing their own particular programmes that rarely overlapped. Only at the Head of the River race was there any evidence of NARA crews competing on the same terms as those from the ARA and, at the event for 1947, three of them – one, Thames Tradesmen's RC, to be a considerable force by the 1970s – were placed in the first division, the leading twenty-five crews.[54]

For the moment, Tugwell's main preoccupation was to find a solution to some of the remaining pre-war problems that were mainly of concern to the NARA. Chief of these was that presented by the residual professionals in the North East and on the Thames. Both groups of oarsmen were anxious to rid themselves of their old labels and Tugwell was very anxious to assist them. He consulted his own body and kept a somewhat suspicious ARA informed of what was happening, although everybody, including the oarsmen, realised that the change might take some time.[55] A crisis of a potentially serious nature occurred not long after the end of the war. Those careful arrangements that Tugwell had designed for the new Northern RA in 1939 were very nearly jeopardised when some of the clubs involved raced at Durham Regatta in 1946 for money prizes. However small the sums involved, those concerned laid themselves open to being called professionals which, in fact, was exactly how the regatta committee regarded them. Once they had realised that it was the intention of the clubs to try to become amateur, the regatta officials altered the terms and conditions of the race for the next year but by then the damage had been done.[56]

Tugwell, once he realised what had happened, was sufficiently alarmed to make a special visit to Newcastle to meet the NRA. Ingenious as ever, he managed to convince almost everybody that the crews involved had raced before the NRA had been able to re-establish its authority and that, had it been properly reconstituted, the oarsmen would not have raced at Durham as professionals and the regatta committee would not have offered money prizes. The slower members of the NRA argued that, since the controlling body had lapsed during the war, they had perforce no choice but to row under the professional banner. Tugwell warned them that to emphasise that particular point could only work to their disadvantage and that they should consider themselves as having been under the NRA since 1939. Any oarsmen, he claimed, who had unwittingly rowed in a professional race since then could apply through the NRA to be reinstated as an amateur and such a decision would be approved by the NARA.[57]

These complex negotiations were in the end accepted by the great bulk of the members of the old professional clubs in the North East. But there were a few, men who had served with great loyalty over the years, who saw the possibility of their being debarred from belonging to their own clubs. For the most part they were too old to row but they had gained much pleasure from their connection with the river and had no wish suddenly to be cut off from a sport they had enjoyed for so long. The Empire RC found a solution that was acceptable to them all, such men being made honorary members on condition that they did not compete. It was a decent and proper way to honour those who were the heirs of Clasper, Chambers and Renforth.[58]

At its meeting in December 1947, the NRA was told that its affiliation had been accepted by the NARA and that Tugwell had at the same time reassured the ARA that these old professional clubs were now genuinely amateur.[59] His anxiety on this score was such that the NARA upheld a complaint in 1949 that the Chester-le-Street RC had rowed at York Regatta with a crew containing men who had earlier won money prizes.[60] The issue was of such a sensitive nature that there was no room for those who tried to break the rules. As it was, it took some time before these clubs were accepted locally as amateurs. It was a matter of some indignation that, whereas regattas outside the North East began to include the clubs on their circulation list, those nearer home appeared to ignore their existence.[61] Nevertheless, these protracted negotiations with the northern clubs became the basis of a similar agreement with the Tradesmen's Rowing Club Association on the Thames. The virtual collapse of professional rowing on that river during the war years meant that Tugwell, with the 1946 business at Durham Regatta very much in his mind, could warn the few of them left to restart their activities cautiously. The Thames men became affiliated to the NARA in 1949 under a rule that any who had lost their amateur status before 1 July 1948 could continue to row on the same conditions as applied to those in the North East.[62]

Tugwell had successfully shepherded these small groups, whose future was likely to be bleak and bankrupt, into the NARA fold. It was an achievement of which he could rightly be proud but he was prepared to extend an equally helping hand to any others who faced difficulties. While acting through the National Fitness Scheme in 1939, he had managed to bring the isolated clubs in Lincolnshire into the NARA. By 1948 the local association there had collapsed but one of its members, Ancholme RC, was one of the few clubs allowed to affiliate directly with the parent body.[63] It was a mark of the improving relations between the ARA and the NARA, largely because Tugwell had been scrupulous in keeping the former informed on these issues, that both jointly in 1952 set their seal of approval on the end of professional rowing in this country by agreeing that anyone who had for any particular reason slipped through the legislative net should be granted a free pardon.[64]

VI

While Tugwell was worrying himself about the fate of the apparently dispossessed, the first steps towards amalgamation were in the process of being taken, the initiative in this instance coming from the ARA. The governing issue was once again foreign competition, as it had been in the shaping of the 1879 Henley rules and the 1884 ARA definition, as well as in part in the 1937 agreement. The British Olympic Committee had agreed that the 1948 games should be held in this country and this meant that the Olympic Regatta would take place at Henley. The prospect of any kind of racing being conducted over those sacred waters by foreigners was something that the ARA and the Henley stewards could only contemplate with distaste. It was decided, therefore, that an approach should be made to FISA about the possibility of joining an organisation that, to date, the ARA had ignored.[65]

During the late summer of 1947, a delegation was sent to the FISA meeting at Lucerne. It consisted of Harcourt Gold, at that time chairman of both Henley and the ARA, David Williams, secretary to Henley Royal

Regatta, Jack Beresford and G. O. Nickalls. As a mark of its firm intent, the ARA persuaded Thames RC to send a coxswainless four and a pair to the European Championships that were taking place at the same time.[66] The NARA was kept fully informed about what was happening since the approach to the FISA was a joint one, in essence a revival of the 1939 idea of a British Rowing Board. On its return, Nickalls reported to the ARA committee on how well they had been received, that the two entries had reached the finals of their events, and that, in principle, the application had been accepted. He told the committee: 'that in order to qualify for admittance to F.I.S.A. it had been necessary to anticipate events and inform F.I.S.A. that the A.R.A. and the N.A.R.A. had become a single body.' He added mischievously that 'the committee might find these sentiments a little premature'.[67] In the circumstances, Nickalls was not taking all that much of a risk since he had ensured that the management of the Olympic Regatta remained in what the committee considered proper hands. At the same time, although he did not immediately admit this, Nickalls had been slightly misleading since it was not until the next year that Great Britain was properly admitted as an ordinary member of FISA and even then the rules of the association had to be waived since no Euro-ᵢ n Championships had been held in this country.[68] No doubt the hosting of two Olympic Regattas was taken into account instead. But from the point of view of the future of domestic rowing, the important consequence of the Lucerne visit was the setting up of a joint ARA and NARA committee, joined later by a Scottish representative, to consider the future of British rowing at international events.[69] It was the first time since the somewhat ineffectual discussions of 1939 that the officials of the two bodies had sat down together to discuss questions of common interest.

There seems little doubt that amalgamation between the two associations would in fact have taken place at some time in the future. Tugwell's message in the 1948 *Almanack* had made clear what his hopes were and Nickalls and Page at the ARA were not unsympathetic. But the decision to join the FISA on behalf of both associations certainly forced the pace. Nickalls' sophistry had effectively disarmed possible critics in the ARA by keeping control of the Olympic Regatta in British hands. But a more important achievement was that he had ensured that there would no longer be any possibility of a retreat into that isolationist frame of mind that had once so characterised the ARA. The victory of the Cambridge eight in the 1951 European Championships effectively ensured that. Nor could there now be any backing down from commitments to the NARA about some form of union. All that remained was to work out the details to the satisfaction of both parties.

Inevitably the newly appointed Joint Committee assumed more importance since it was the only body where all concerned could meet formally together. It took a number of soundings, including a dinner held after the 1948 Head of the River Race to which were invited R. D. Burnell, former Oxford blue, future Olympic gold medallist and editor of the *Almanack*, George Rogers of Australia and H. A. Barry, the old professional sculling champion of the world. Informal discussions, the exchange of ideas and the indication of possible areas of difficulty were an important part of the process. The *Almanack* felt the dinner was sufficiently worth reporting since 'it further cemented the good relations between the two associations'.[70] Tugwell was encouraged enough by all this to write to the ARA stating that the issue of amalgamation ought to be placed on the agenda of both parties and the Joint Committee was formally asked to investigate the matter.[71]

The result was the production in March 1949 of a confidential report by Charles Tugwell and David Williams, the Henley secretary. It laid out clearly the differences between the two assocations, particularly the far more representative nature of the NARA council and the degree of autonomy which was allowed to its constituent associations. It indicated the greater membership of the ARA – some 16,500 compared with just under 6,500 – and the fact that financially the NARA was the poorer of the two bodies.[72] Far more important were its proposals for the future. On the assumption that the Scottish ARA might wish to join, the recommended name was the British ARA and its objectives would be to encourage and protect amateur rowing, to affiliate to the relevant foreign bodies, and to organise crews for international competition.[73] The report envisaged a potential membership of some 24,000 and argued that the clubs should be grouped into locally autonomous divisions that would be arranged so that they would embrace the former NARA associations. Each division would be responsible for its own finances but would be expected to collect the subscriptions payable to the parent body.[74] Finally, there would be a council of thirty which would be far more like the existing NARA arrangements than the unrepresentative ARA system. Only the provision of one delegate each to OUBC, CUBC and Leander paid lip-service to the strength of the nominating group on the ARA committee.[75]

It is not at all clear how much consultation there was on this report. The provincial meeting of the ARA, for example, always a useful sounding-board, does not appear to have discussed it, although its chairman, S. H. Johnson, was privy to the discussions.[76] Nevertheless, the ARA committee in June 1950 expressed its general approval, the only note of caution being a financial one since it was felt that new organisation would need a substantially larger income than the report had suggested – £3,000 per year as against £650. It was concluded that both bodies should 'put their houses in order' without, in fact, specifying in what way and that the question should be reopened at a later date.[77] It all sounded a little lukewarm and lacking in enthusiasm.

The NARA had one specific problem, its legal status as an incorporated body, and it was feared that this might prove something of an obstacle to amalgamation but in practice a solution was found without very much difficulty.[78] The real dilemma seemed to lie with the ARA, since it was being asked to accept what was a fundamental change in its structure. The granting of greater freedom to the local divisions was a concession to NARA usage but in fact was not much different from the way in which the local ARA associations had been allowed to work out regatta dates except in one crucial respect. The suggestion that the new divisions should be given considerable financial independence seemed to clash with the ARA's view that the parent body would need a larger income. But this was to prove a small matter compared with the report's radical reshaping of the central council of the new organisation. What was being asked of the ARA was that a select group of clubs, each with a privileged position, should surrender rights that dated back to the origins of the ARA. These clubs were the direct heirs of Selwyn, Shadwell and Egan and they found the suggested changes unpalatable. Members of the NARA had recognised that this was likely to prove a major stumbling block. The minutes of the Northern RA cautioned against too hasty a reaction on the issue: 'We are working on the more democratic lines, whilst the A.R.A. appears to be working on lines handed down from father to son.'[79]

This obstacle of what to do with the original nominating clubs of the ARA effectively closed the discussion for the next four years. For a moment it looked as if the ARA might turn in on itself again. But while the most powerful group on the committee clung obstinately to its special position, its representatives from the elite clubs suddenly began to look vulnerable. The international successes following the end of the war had proved to be a false dawn. At the 1952 Olympic Regatta, there were no medals for Great Britain and at the 1954 Empire and Commonwealth Games, no English crew won an event. At Henley, Soviet boats appeared, winning the Grand in 1954, the Stewards as well as the Goblets in 1954 and 1955. Early in 1954, *The Rowing Magazine* blisteringly attacked the ARA over its selection policy, especially at a time when it was collecting funds on a compulsory basis from club oarsmen to support international competition.[80] It returned to the attack six months later over attempts to find crews to go to the Empire and Commonwealth Games. Leander apparently was not good enough, London RC was never approached, enquiries were made around the Cambridge colleges, others would not go, while Pengwern RC from Shrewsbury, winners of the West of England Vase and of the coxed four championship was not considered.[81] The editor of the magazine was not privy to the deliberations of the selection committee and no doubt much of what was written was based on hearsay and gossip. But it was an angry indictment, betraying frustration and lack of confidence, and, at a time when there were still problems and shortages at club level, unlikely to improve the image of the sport or the morale of its oarsmen.[82]

This was not a matter that Tugwell raised when he reminded the ARA in January 1954 that amalgamation was still on the agenda of both associations. To have done so would have seemed like an intrusion into private grief. Instead he simply informed the ARA that his own body was in the process of settling its own particular problems and, by implication, asking the ARA what progress it was making with its own. G. O. Nickalls was acutely conscious of the way his own committee was dragging its feet and he firmly told its members that 'we should show rather more readiness to understand the N.A.R.A. point of view than had been evident in the past.'[83] But three months later the ARA minutes still indicated the degree of reluctance that existed over the question of the nominating group of clubs.[84]

Both Nickalls and Page were in a difficult and unenviable position with a committee that was clearly in an odd frame of mind – obstinate, proud, a little sullen about the shape of things to come. Since the war, the ARA committee had abandoned a number of ideals and practices that in earlier years it would have condemned. It had allowed those who worked 'in and about boats' to compete as amateurs, it had agreed that those rowing abroad would not jeopardise their amateur status by accepting legitimate expenses and it had accepted that, provided he received no money prize, any amateur could compete in the race for the Doggetts' Coat and Badge.[85] At the same time it had begun to assume new obligations. For example, during 1952, it was forced to accept responsibility for the Women's ARA in order to meet the requirements of FISA, a body already working on the assumption that there was only one controlling body for rowing in this country.[86] Aware of all these contradictions and that the situation was potentially embarrassing, Page persuaded his committee to respond to Tugwell's suggestion that a draft constitution might be drawn up for a British ARA.[87] By October the discussions were proceeding reasonably smoothly. Already it was emerging that some clubs, anxious for amalgamation, were joining both associations.[88] The final draft was elastic enough to embrace most of the NARA regattas and championships and so designed as to encourage its clubs to join the new organisation. At the October meeting of the ARA, when these fresh ideas were presented, there was a further item calling for serious reconsideration of international selection procedures following the Empire and Commonwealth Games. Some obdurate figures could apparently see no connection between the two issues and, by a small majority, the draft constitution was rejected. Instead the NARA was offered a form of extraordinary association with some co-opted members on the ARA committee. The NARA council in its turn refused to accept what it saw as a condescending approach.[89]

By the May 1955 meeting, the obstinate element in the ARA was still trying to defend its position, but in fact the narrowness of the vote the previous October had indicated that the unity of the privileged group was breaking.[90] The NARA's immediate refusal to accept what it saw as a demeaning alternative, followed by the abject failure of any British crews to reach any finals of that year's European Championships, seemed to be enough to bring the diehards to their senses. Page clearly realised that amalgamation was now achievable and, sensing the mood of his committee, encouraged Tugwell to circulate details of the proposals for the new constitution to all NARA clubs and associations during the early autumn. On 22 October, the NARA agreed to what was in fact its demise. Two weeks later, the ARA committee accepted the inevitable.[91]

The NARA had sacrificed itself, as it was bound to do, to the senior and more powerful body. At their annual meeting in November 1955, the representatives of the provincial ARA clubs applauded Charles Tugwell and his council, echoing J. H. Page's view 'that everyone felt the strongest admiration and gratitude to them for their action in the cause of national rowing'.[92] From 1 January 1956, the new ARA welcomed applications for affiliation from all former NARA clubs in England and Wales, additional provincial divisions were created, the old NARA associations were reborn as regatta councils and the ARA agreed to promote a new national championship, using the NARA trophies. Two members of the NARA, one of them Charles Tugwell, became members of the new committee. Initially it looked as if the contentious issue of the nominating clubs had hardly been tampered with. Kingston RC, Molesey BC and Twickenham RC lost their right to a member each and had to be content with one between the three of them. The others remained as before. But, in practice, the balance on the committee had been crucially altered. The old Group I, the nominating group, dropped from seventeen to fourteen members, while the rest increased from eleven in 1955 to fifteen after amalgamation, to be enhanced by three more once the coastal clubs joined after recovering from their jubilee celebrations.[93] This was in fact a significant victory for Tugwell and the NARA standpoint, as well as for the smaller and the provincial clubs. Although at first sight it looked as if the NARA, in agreeing to its disappearance, had suffered most, it was in fact the praetorian guard and its representatives who were now hemmed in. Some of the smaller clubs recognised the full significance of the change. 'The concessions,' stated the secretary of the Furnivall Scullers, 'which have been made by the A.R.A. go far beyond what we had dared to hope for a few seasons ago.[94]

VII

It cannot always have been obvious, particularly in the provinces, what immediate gains were to be expected from amalgamation. Officially the absorption of the NARA went smoothly enough. Nevertheless there was a danger that some clubs might decide in the new circumstances to remain unaffiliated. It needed the threat that regattas under ARA rules should only accept entries from those in the assocation to undermine that particular tendency.[95] The successful NARA championships did not prosper under the new order and in the end it was agreed to discontinue them until a suitable course could be found or built.[96] Nor was there much scope for developing the former NARA associations under a different guise and several, like Tugwell's carefully nurtured Northern Rowing Association, decided to disband themselves.[97]

Nevertheless, within a decade, clubs and regattas began to thrive and it is probable that the name of the NARA was virtually forgotten. In 1965, entries at Henley were over 200 and topped 150 at a number of others, Bedford, Marlow, Reading, Wallingford and St Neots, the latter once an old NARA event,[98] Others found, especially among junior and novice crews, that special arrangements were needed to cope with the large numbers anxious to compete.[99] Some former NARA clubs, most notably Thames Tradesmen's RC, began to figure prominently among the leading clubs in the country. In 1963 the Women's ARA was absorbed into the ARA and rowing began to attract women equally with men to the genuine benefit of clubs and regattas.[100] But it was rare at first to see all this vigour being transformed into success at international level.

A spate of letters in *The Rowing Magazine* during the autumn of 1956 testified to the fear that, in spite of amalgamation, old habits and practices might continue to the detriment of rowing. Some of the suggestions were sensible enough, demanding an investigation into the methods and techniques of more successful European crews or urging the provision of a modern multi-lane course. Others deplored the continued intrusion of the past, the sterile arguments between the upholders of orthodoxy and the approach of Steve Fairbairn or what they saw as the restraining influence of the two universities and of Leander.[101] For the main part all this was unfair to the ARA as it wrestled with its inadequate resources over the issue of how to revitalise rowing both domestically and at an international level. A delicate balancing act was needed – and not always achieved – since too great an emphasis on one could lead to criticism that the other was being ignored. In practice, many of the initiatives were intended to help all participants, whatever their standards and skills. The appointment in 1964 of the first of several professional national coaches was intended not just to improve rowing techniques and training but to create a climate of opinion open to fresh ideas. This was further reinforced by the provision of weekend coaching courses that were, in turn, to lead to a more structured approach to the sport.[102] The long search for a suitable site for a modern rowing course ended when the National Water Sports Centre was opened at Holme Pierrepont, a joint venture between the Nottingham County Council and the Sports Council, enabling genuine National Championships to be held from 1972 onwards.[103] All these were solid achievements, available to those clubs prepared to take advantage of them, essential for international success.

By the late 1960s and the 1970s, a number of clubs, the University of London, Barn Cottage and the Tideway Scullers School – the latter two virtually privately inspired elite squads – were indicating that Britain could achieve success abroad. The introduction during the early 1970s of a genuine national squad, under the coaching of a former Czech oarsman, Bohumil Janousek, provided the breakthrough. In 1974, at the

World Championships at Lucerne, the British eight unexpectedly won the silver medal. Two years later, at the Olympic Regatta in Canada, basically the same eight repeated the performance. To be second in the world might not have satisfied an earlier generation but, by the 1970s, the physical demands imposed on competitors, especially those who were amateurs in the full sense, was such that medals of any kind indicated real excellence. Those twin silver medals marked the end of some twenty years of argument about the future of rowing in this country. They foreshadowed further success, including gold medals at the Olympics, the World Championships and at Lightweight and Junior levels. 1974 and 1976 represented, perhaps a little tardily, the hopes expressed in 1937 that one day Great Britain could produce a genuinely representative crew. The crews concerned were drawn from two clubs, Leander and Thames Tradesmen, one the elite of the old praetorian guard, the other once a member of the NARA. Not so many years earlier, they would not have been allowed to appear together in the same boat.

The international dimension had often been a cause of argument as well as an impulse towards change. If one of the undercurrents that finally forced through amalgamation in 1956 was the lack of success in foreign competition, the remedy was, in fact, to take some years before it was seen to be effective. When it came, however, it was a sound recovery, one that was based on safely established foundations. Although those crews aspiring to row internationally tended to be centred on the Thames and to a lesser extent at Nottingham, their credentials are now a good deal more widely-based than was the case a few decades ago. At the same time, the ARA tried to reflect many of these changes in its own organisation and in 1967–8 it critically reduced the voting power of the privileged caucus in its midst. The various groups and divisions were reformed and in the process the old Group I – the nominating clubs – disappeared. OUBC, CUBC, Leander, London RC and Thames RC retained one representative each, a small minority amongst all the others. J. H. Page justified this small degree of ancient prerogative, stating, somewhat wistfully and nostalgically, that 'because of their history, the part they have played and the part they are still capable of playing, few will think that this is a disproportionate share'.[104]

These five clubs were the irreducible core of those that had shaped the course and pattern of English rowing for well over a century. Their influence both at home and abroad has been immense, profoundly affecting the nature of the sport. Behind a mask of often crusty conservatism, they set high standards that they believed were worth preserving. At the heart of their creed, as befitted the heirs of Selwyn, Shadwell and Egan, was a deep belief in the virtues of amateurism. Their greatest fault was their failure to realise that others, often less privileged than themselves, could share similar beliefs. This obstinate misjudgement was to condemn English rowing, for the best part of seventy years, to a degree of sectarian division that convinced many who saw the sport from outside that it was essentially an exclusive affair for a select few. Nevertheless, by striking such a posture, this small group forced their critics squarely to face the implications of what was meant by the term amateur. At the same time, they themselves came to recognise some virtue in becoming less rigid and narrow. Throughout the long debate, expediency was often confused with principle to the extent that significant numbers of clubs and regattas stood aloof from the bewildering and, on occasions, disagreeable debate. But, whatever the motives may have been at a particular time, so finely honed did the concept of an amateur become that rowing still remains, for the great majority of its participants, one of the few sports that still honours its tradition and meaning.

By the 1970s and the 1980s there was evidence of some greater degree of flexibility of attitude and, in a few cases, it might seem as if the amateur code was being seriously compromised. Professional coaches were being employed by the ARA as well as by the universities at Oxford, Cambridge and London. Sponsorship was being eagerly sought at all levels and in 1988 FISA allowed the best international oarsmen, like the better-known athletes, to establish trust funds to assist with training in an increasingly time-consuming and competitive sport.[105] All this might suggest a new beginning and an abandonment of long cherished but dated notions. In another sense, it is a reminder of one more important tradition in English rowing, one that a hundred years earlier had focused public attention on the Thames and particularly on the Tyne. But in those days professional rowing had been able to attract a sufficient number of interested sponsors and large if often unruly crowds of spectators.

Such conditions no longer exist. More than ever international competition at so many different levels – senior, junior, women, lightweight – exercises its influence and to cope successfully with its demands means an amplitude of resource that currently does not exist. The problem is that rowing is not a popular spectator sport and has little attraction to the general public or to the media. The many who flock annually to Henley Royal Regatta do so because it is as much a part of society's summer scene as a rowing occasion. Attendance at the National Championships on a multi-lane course attracts far fewer. Television, that has transformed a number of sports and games such as athletics, show-jumping and snooker, is unlikely to have a similar effect on rowing. Except occasionally in sculling and other small boats, rowing rarely produces its public heroes and the nature of the sport in any case discourages the adulation of the individual. It fortunately means that, even with the setting up of trust funds for a limited number of oarsmen, they are unlikely to be manipulated by agents in the way that often happens in athletics, attracting controversy and publicity. Apart from the Boat Race – itself a paradoxical legacy from a more privileged age – rowing rarely commands much attention. It is an ironic comment on the strength of those values advanced so many years ago by Selwyn, Shadwell and Egan that a private match between two universities should still remain in the public mind as rowing's most important occasion.

Notes

1 *The Proceedings of the First Conference of the Amateur Rowing Association*, 1927, p. 11.
2 C. S. Bell, *Derby Rowing Club – The First Hundred years 1879–1979* (Derby, 1979), p. 17.
3 John Allen, 'Reading Regattas', *The British Rowing Almanack*, 1964, pp. 192–6.
4 *The Almanack*, 1924, p. 195.
5 *Ibid.*, 1934, p. 107.
6 Weybridge RC, *Minutes*, 2 November 1925, 1 July 1935.
7 Tideway Boxing Day Charity Regatta, *Minutes*, 9 November 1925, 18 April, 24 October, 17 December 1929.
8 *The Times*, 12 June 1937.
9 NARA, *Handbook for 1937*, p. 6.
10 H. Cleaver, *A History of Rowing* (London, 1957), p. 148; *Hansard – Parliamentary Debates*, 322, 7 April 1937, pp. 236–7.
11 Britain won a gold in the double sculls and a silver in the coxswainless fours. Germany, on the other hand, won medals in all the available events – five golds, a silver and a bronze.
12 *The Times*, 10 April 1937.
13 *Ibid.*
14 The delegates were from the ARA: C. M. Pitman (OUBC and Leander), C. T. Steward (Leander), F. F. Saunders (Quintin BC), The Hon. John Freemantle (CUBC, Leander and Secretary of the ARA); from the NARA: T. S. Charles (Thames ARA), W. V. Chilvers (Norwich ARA), G. T. Launchbury (Oxford ARA), H. H. Stride (Hants and Dorset ARA), C. B. S. Tugwell (Secretary,

NARA). In the event E. A. Samuels (Folkestone RC) took the place of Chilvers. Cleaver, *A History of Rowing*, pp. 142–3; *The Almanack*, 1937, p. 109.

15 Cleaver, *A History of Rowing*, pp. 143–5.

16 *The Almanack*, 1938, p. 105.

17 Cleaver, *A History of Rowing*, pp. 145–6; *The Almanack*, 1938, pp. 105–7; NARA, *Handbook for 1938*, pp. 20–1; Henley Royal Regatta, *Minutes*, 'Special meeting', 10 June 1937.

18 *The Times*, 12 June 1937.

19 Cleaver, *A History of Rowing*, p. 148; NARA, *Handbook for 1938*, pp. 20–1.

20 ARA, *Minutes*, 27 February 1938.

21 *Ibid.*, 24 April 1939.

22 NARA, *Handbook for 1938*, pp. 21–2; ARA, *Minutes*, 11 February, 31 October 1938.

23 *The Almanack*, 1938, Preface, pp. xiv–xv.

24 NARA, *Handbook for 1939*, p. 20.

25 Weybridge RC, *Minutes*, 2, 11 November 1938, 11 January, 11 April, 2 May, 6 June 1939.

26 Tees ABC, *Minutes*, 1 April, 3 May 1938, 5 April 1939 *Annual Report, 1939*.

27 Evesham R.C., *Minutes*, 8 April, 27 July 1938, 24 March, 12 May, 23 June, 7 July, 21 July, 4 August 1939.

28 ARA, *Minutes*, 1939 – Insert: 'Schemes for the improvement of rowing facilities in connection with the National Fitness Campaign'.

29 Empire R.C., *Minutes*, 'Special meeting', 23 October 1939.

30 Meeting of northern professional clubs, *Minutes*, Northern Rowing Association, 21 November 1938.

31 Northern Rowing Association, *Minutes*, 28 April 1939.

32 *Newcastle Evening Chronicle*, 5 May 1939.

33 Empire RC, *Minutes*, 4 May 1939; Cambois R.C., *Minutes*, 15 May 1939.

34 *Newcastle Evening Chronicle*, 5 June 1939.

35 W. A. Locan, *The Agecroft Story – The First Hundred Years of Agecroft R.C., 1861–1960* (Salford, 1960), pp. 49–51.

36 Evesham RC, *Minutes*, 30 May 1941, 20 March 1942, 12 February 1943, 23 March 1945.

37 Weybridge RC, *Minutes*, 5 March, 15 October 1941, 8 July, 26 August 1942.

38 Empire RC, *Minutes*, 8 May, October (no day) 1941.

39 Furnivall Sculling Club, *Annual Report*, March 1948.

40 Tyne ARC, *Minutes*, 7 February 1946.

41 Tees ABC, *Minutes*, 2 March 1940, 10 April 1943, 28 December 1944, 10 May 1945, 3, 9 May 1946.

42 *Exeter Express and Echo*, 15 April 1964.

43 Falcon RC, *Minutes*, 14 December 1945, 10 April 1947, 19 April 1949.

44 Locan, *The Agecroft Story*, pp. 52–6.

45 Furnivall Sculling Club, *Minutes*, 'Annual Report', March 1948.

46 Empire RC, *Minutes*, 14 October 1946.

47 *Ibid.*, *Notes* in souvenir programme of Tyne United RC's annual dance, 26 November 1948.

48 Tyne A.R.C., *Minutes*, 8 May 1946, 16 January, 1 May 1947.

49 Tees A.R.C., *Minutes*, 10, 24 May 1946, 19 January, 3 May 1948.

50 *The Almanack*, 1949, p. 19; Provincial Committee of the ARA, November 1952, p. 4, November 1957, pp. 6–7.
51 Provincial Committee of the ARA, November 1952, pp. 3–4. Coxed fours were introduced at Henley in 1963.
52 *Joint Report of ARA and NARA*, 30 March 1949, s. 3–4.
53 C. B. S. Tugwell, 'ARA and NARA – the differences between them', *The Almanack*, 1948, pp. 25–6.
54 *The Almanack*, 1948, p. 57.
55 NARA, *Minutes*, 20 November 1948; ARA, *Minutes*, 18 November 1947, 20 December 1948; Empire RC, *Minutes*, 28 March 1947.
55 Durham Regatta, *Minutes*, 30 April 1947.
57 Northern Rowing Association, *Minutes*, 7 December 1946, 8 March 1947, 29 May 1948; *The Almanack*, 1948, pp. 17–8.
58 Empire RC, *Minutes*, 6 June 1947.
59 NARA, *Minutes*, 15 November 1947; Northern Rowing Association, *Minutes*, 13 December 1947.
60 NARA, *Minutes*, 26 March 1949.
61 Northern Rowing Association, *Minutes*, 29 May 1948.
62 NARA, *Minutes*, 26 March 1949.
63 NARA, *Handbook for 1939*, p. 19 and *The Almanack*, 1948, p. 32.
64 NARA, *Minutes*, 18 October 1952.
65 ARA, *Minutes*, 27 May 1946.
66 *The Almanack*, 1948, p. 9.
67 ARA, *Minutes*, 6 October 1947.
68 *The Almanack*, 1950, p. 16.
69 ARA, *Minutes*, 6 October 1947; NARA, *Minutes*, 20 November 1947.
70 *The Almanack* 1950, p. 16.
71 ARA, *Minutes*, 5 October 1948.
72 *Joint Report of ARA and NARA*, s. 3–4.
73 *Ibid.*, s. 13, 14.
74 *Ibid.*, s. 17–20, 23, 24.
75 *Ibid.*, s. 21.
76 ARA, *Minutes*, 20 December 1948.
77 *Ibid.*, 12 June 1950.
78 *Joint Report of ARA and NARA*, s. 10.
79 Northern Rowing Association, *Minutes*, 20 November 1948.
80 *Rowing Magazine*, January 1954.
81 *Ibid.*, June 1954.
82 *The Almanack*, 1955, pp. 8–9 where the review of 1954 draws attention to the continued financial difficulties of many clubs and the problems arising from the high costs of transport.
83 ARA, *Minutes*, 25 January 1954.
84 NARA, *Minutes*, 2 April 1954.
85 ARA, *Minutes*, 12 February 1946, 1 April, 16 June 1947, 12 June 1950.
86 *The Almanack*, 1953, p. 17.
87 NARA, *Minutes*, 2 April 1954; ARA, *Minutes*, 8 April 1954.
88 The 1949 NARA list included the following in both associations – Boston, Military College of Science, Eton Vikings, Barnes, Burway, Harrodian,

Linden, Metropolitan Police, Panther, Thames, Tradesmen and Weybridge.
89 ARA, *Minutes*, 20 October 1954; NARA, *Minutes*, 30 October 1954.
90 ARA, *Minutes*, 5 May 1955.
91 Furnivall Sculling Club, *Minutes*, 17 September 1955; NARA, *Minutes*, 22 October 1955; ARA, *Minutes*, 3 November 1955.
92 *Provincial Committee of the ARA*, 1955, p. 7.
93 *The Almanack*, 1957, p. 6.
94 Furnivall Sculling Club, *Minutes*, 17 September 1955.
95 Provincial Committee of the ARA, 1956, p. 11.
96 *Ibid.*, p. 5 and for 1957, p. 4; ARA, *Minutes*, 17 October 1957; *The Almanack*, 1966, p. 42.
97 Northern Rowing Association, *Minutes*, 17 March 1956.
98 K. Osborne, *Boat Racing in Britain, 1715–1975*, (London, 1975), pp. 60–1; *The Almanack*, 1966, p. 42.
99 Durham Regatta, *Minutes*, 17 June 1959.
100 *The Almanack*, 1964, pp. 244–5.
101 *Rowing Magazine*, October 1956.
102 ARA, *Minutes*, 26 October 1960, 17 July 1961, 29 January 1962, 15 October 1963; *The Almanack*, 1964, pp. 243–4.
103 Osborne, *Boat-Racing*, pp. 61–2.
104 *The Almanack*, 1968, p. 263.
105 ARA, *Rowers and Money* (London, 1989).

Appendix I – Boats and style

Boats, during the early nineteenth century, came in all sorts of shapes and sizes, whether they were used for work or for pleasure. Barges, keelboats and foy boats shared the river with the funny, the wherry, the cutter, the ran-dan and the gig. Many of these boats could be used with various types of rig. The ordinary Thames wherry, normally built for one or two pairs of sculls or for two oars, could on occasions be extended to four or eight oars, one of the latter, belonging to Lord Castlereagh, existing in 1840. Similar variations were to be found among cutters and gigs, some being constructed for four, six or eight oars, the last type being used for the first Boat Race in 1829.[1] But boats with ten oars existed at Eton and Westminster, while London RC had a twelve-oar during the 1860s that was used to pace the university crews at Putney.[2]

Why the eight-oar should have emerged as the largest of the racing boats is far from clear. Drinkwater and Sanders have argued that it was but natural to copy the eight-oared barges of the City companies of eighteenth century London.[3] Byrne and Churchill have sensibly pointed out that, especially in the days of fixed seat rowing, anything with more than eight oars would, at pace, have had some difficulty in clearing its own wash and the puddles of the previous stroke.[4] It may well be that the answer is more prosaic. By doubling successively from a single scull to a pair, and from a pair to a four, the neat result produced an eight. To have gone any further would have been to build a monstrosity.

By the early 1860s the modern racing boat had effectively begun to emerge. The anonymous author on rowing in *The Manual of British Rural Sports*, published in 1861, confined the wherry, gig and such-like boats to 'watermen's purposes or for pleasure-parties' and stated that, except for those learning to row, they were 'quite exploded as racing boats'.[5] In fact a specially designed wager-wherry had emerged by the 1830s, a single sculling boat, narrow at the beam but with exaggerated flared sides for the rowlocks. It continued to be used well towards the end of the century in the Doggett's and other apprentice races as well as by some amateur regattas, including Henley in its early days.[6] At their best, these wager boats could apparently weigh as little as twenty-five pounds which, if true, was astoundingly light for clinker-built boats.[7] The fairly massive spread of the gunwales on such boats gives some indication of the amount of thought that went into the business of increasing leverage. The oarsmen on the Oxford boat of 1829, essentially a derivative of the naval gig like the Exeter College, Oxford boat of 1824, sat as far over from their rowlocks as possible for the same reason.[8] It was a problem that exercised a number of oarsmen during the early part of the nineteenth century, including some of those active on the Tyne.

The provision of a crude outrigger may well have been considered in various parts of the country. It must be doubted whether the earliest attempts were any better than the flared sides of the wager-wherries, although the students at Durham, during the mid-1830s, found the normally constructed gigs built in the south slower than the boats with riggers that they acquired locally.[9] The Tyne seems to have encouraged some experiments with riggers during the late 1820s. Anthony Brown of Ouseburn fixed wooden blocks to the side of *The Diamond* for his race against *The Fly* of Scotswood in 1828, while Frank Emmett of Dent's Hole, after first using wood, fitted iron riggers to *The Eagle* in 1830. Harry Clasper is credited with having improved and perfected these rudimentary structures but, as far as is known, did not fit them to any of his own racing boats before the early 1840s, by which time a similar development had taken place in Dublin.[10] Rowe and Pitman confirm the experience of the undergraduates at Durham, pointing out that the outrigger became popular in the north long before it was accepted in the south.[11] But the reason for this may be simply that the boat-builders on the Thames were perfecting the old-fashioned cutters and gigs into fine and successful racing boats. Clasper, although in the process of building during 1842 his revolutionary four, *The Five Brothers*, was nevertheless forced to use his old boat, the *St Agnes*, for his race against Coombes' crew. The latter's boat was much the lighter, weighing 160 pounds, and was described as 'a beautiful model of this class of running boat'. Both craft were clinker-built and, according to the same report, 'rowed off the gunwale'; in other words, neither had outriggers. A much later description of *St Agnes*, written in 1861, suggests that, although the heavier of the two boats, it was in fact outrigged, a comment that hardly squares with the earlier criticism 'that the whole of the crew sitting on one side could not upset her'.[12] But the main point is that the victorious Coombes crew were using what seems to have been a remarkable example of the Thames boat-builders' skill, a conventional enough craft but one of considerable speed and lightness. This was certainly the contemporary defence of Clasper's defeat. The correspondent of the *Tyne Mercury* concluded that: 'although the men of the Tyne have lost the race, it is not to be inferred from that that they have lost their honour as oarsmen . . . Let their friends furnish them with a proper boat and we are very much mistaken if the result of another contest is not different.'[13]

The Five Brothers was that boat. Clasper's crew first used it at the Tyne Regatta in August 1843 and then, in June 1844, won with it on the first day at the Royal Thames Regatta. It was built of mahogany, just over thirty-seven feet long, two feet at its widest point, and with iron outriggers. It was also keelless, the keel being inside the boat and the skin being of shell construction. Some twenty years later, the *Almanack* recalled that: 'she created much speculation and excitement among the Thames watermen. Her construction was quite revolutionary to their settled notions of racing vessels, and it was believed it would be impossible to row her steadily, as she was as round in the bottom as the section of half a gun barrel.'[14] At the same regatta, Clasper carried off the main sculling prize and his boat, according to Woodgate, was the first of its kind to be fitted with outriggers.[15] It is far from clear whether this was also a keelless boat but it seems probable that the two that were used in a sculling match on the Tyne in December 1844 were. Clasper's boat was described as 'a perfect model in form, almost a toy, more fit as an ornament for a parlour than a boat to row in' and, suggestive that it was in fact a derivative of his four, as 'the beau ideal of his four-oared gig, *The Five Brothers*.[16] That Coombes, his opponent, turned up with a boat of only forty-three pounds, six less than that of the Tyne oarsman, seems to indicate that his too was of similar construction.[17] Who built this boat is not clear. William Pocock, a useful Thames professional, at one time claimed that Clasper had stolen the idea of the shell, keelless boat from him and perhaps he may have been responsible. That lighter boats were being constructed seems indisputable. In April 1844 Robert Newell, a London waterman, beat four Belgians rowing in a gig in a race from Ostend to Bruges. His sculling boat, the property of a certain Captain Tollemack and built by Wentzell and Cownden of Lambeth, amazed the Belgians who were 'stunned at her lightness and beauty of construction'.[18] In the same year, Samuel Wolsencroft of the Civil Engineers

College, built himself an outrigged sculling boat and tried to make the skin out of one single piece of wood. Unfortunately he was unable to bend the wood sufficiently without splitting it.[19]

The best of the professionals almost certainly adapted to the new type of boat fairly quickly. How willingly or successfully the amateurs did remains uncertain. James Wallace, an old Tyne amateur, recalled that Talkin Tarn had a keelless four of Clasper's in 1853 and that Tyne ARC in the same year bought a similar boat from Robert Jewett, another Tyne builder. He also claimed to have rowed in a keelless pair, built before 1850. His suggestion that Exeter College acquired a keelless eight in 1846 seems unprobable and it may be that, in his old age, he was remembering that college's acquisition from Royal Chester of the Matthew Taylor eight, ten years later.[20] But some amateurs, like Wolsencroft, were prepared to experiment even if some of their ideas were unsuccessful or on occasions simply bizarre. Dr Furnivall, not one to indulge in the frivolous even while an undergraduate at Trinity Hall, claimed he had built the first two narrow wager-boats ever constructed in 1844, aided by Jack Beesley of St John's, but unfortunately he never gave any firmer information.[21] The next year, with the encouragement of their employer, some brewery men at North Shields built 'a two-oared skiff of block tin, with air boxes' that was no more successful than the sculling boat constructed, in 1847, by W. Austen Ashe along the lines of the market boats he had seen in Ceylon.[22]

Nor were those amateurs who adopted some of the innovations always good advertisements for their use. In 1845, J. W. Conant of St John's College, Oxford, entered for the Diamonds at Henley in an outrigged boat. In his first race he so outclassed his opponent that, according to *Bell's Life*, the latter 'fairly turned round on his thwart to see what had become of Mr. Conant' but, in the final, he in his turn was badly beaten, coming last of three.[23] Others did not always have the courage of their convictions. In 1841 the Oxford crew used a keeled but carvel-built boat, the planks being arranged to produce a smooth surface. But, following their defeat in the Boat Race, Oxford decided not to pursue the idea any further the next year.[24] Cambridge, apparently, had an outrigged boat built for them in eight days for the 1845 Boat Race but, in the end, decided not to use the craft.[25] Such alarms and fears were, however, beginning to be allayed. Partly-outrigged gigs were making their appearance – the riggers being at stroke and bow – and then, confirming the importance of the development, both crews used fully outrigged boats in the 1846 Boat Race.[26] OUBC began to come to terms with the new type of boat when, in winning the Stewards at Henley in 1852, they used a Clasper-built keelless four, the first time an amateur crew had been seen in this type of boat at the regatta.[27]

The eight produced for Cambridge in 1845 was apparently sixty feet long.[28] During the 1850s, the tendency to build longer boats was largely an attempt to reduce what was known at the time as longitudinal oscillation, a problem that appears to have obsessed a number of oarsmen and boat-builders. It was an issue raised again following the introduction of the slide and, in spite of the arguments of Dr Warre that the problem was of no importance, some eights during the 1870s were as long as sixty-three to sixty-six feet.[29] The question of building eights to such an excessive length had, in fact, been raised slightly earlier during the 1850s, in particular by the famous boat built for Royal Chester RC in 1856 by Matthew Taylor, a member of another well-known Tyne waterman's family. This boat, in which the Chester club won both the Grand and the Ladies Plate at Henley, was an object of curiosity and interest from the very beginning. It was fully outrigged as well as keelless and apparently the crew, in spite of two famous victories at one regatta, found it difficult to control.[30] Many years later one of its members, James Fairrie, denied the charge, claiming that Taylor thought its pace would be increased if the work was set as low as possible. He seems to have overdone the experiment since 'some of the crew had difficulty in clearing their knees and flipped the water on the feather every stroke'.[31] It may be that this is the correct explanation of what most on-lookers had regarded at the time as very untidy rowing, surprising in the case of the Chester men since they had the previous year won both the Stewards and the Wyfolds in a Taylor keelless four and, apart from their victories, their performance had attracted no particular comment.

But what, in fact, seemed to arouse most controversy about Taylor's 1856 eight was not that it was outrigged and keelless but that it had a peculiar shape. Fairrie claimed that Taylor was trying to model his boat on that of the porpoise, full forward and fine aft. Certainly her broadest beam appears to have been near the bows and she was a great deal shorter than the traditional eights of that time, being about fifty-five feet in length. G. C. Bourne refused to believe that someone, who had no knowledge of theoretical principles, could have designed by himself a boat of such revolutionary design since, he argued, what made it distinctive was not that it was keelless but that it was short and broad. Instead, Bourne felt that the Chester stroke, J. B. Littledale, a member of a Liverpool shipping family and as such probably aware of some of the new ideas being developed in ship design at that time, must have played an important part in making the decisions about the shape. Bourne advanced the view that the 1856 eight was in effect an attempt to adapt the lines of the *Great Eastern* to use in a racing boat.[32] It is of course impossible to adjudicate on this issue. But Bourne's dismissal of Taylor as simply a skilled craftsmen carrying out orders seems a little cruel given the considerable ingenuity and willingness to experiment of contemporary Tyne professionals. It seems hard to believe that Taylor's role in all this was simply that of a capable cabinet-maker.

The 1856 boat was bought by R. W. Risley of Exeter College, Oxford, and his college crew went Head of the River in her, in 1857, as well as winning the Ladies Plate. Oxford also used a Taylor boat for the 1857 Boat Race, purchased out of his own pocket by the president, A. P. Lonsdale. Oxford rowed a practice course in the boat in 19 minutes 50 seconds, a remarkable time in a fixed seat boat. They won the Boat Race convincingly and Taylor is said to have remarked that, had Cambridge used one of his boats, they would have won too.[33] At six, in the 1857 Oxford crew, was Warre who immediately became convinced about the merits of its shape and, once he became a master of Eton, had a similar boat built by Taylor in which the school won the Ladies Plate six times between 1864 and 1870.[34]

By the 1870s it seems probable that most clubs were adopting the keelless type of boat for their best crews and had accepted the outrigger. Whether or not eights should be long or short appears to have been an enduring controversy that depended in the main on the whims of coaches and oarsmen. The most successful of the professionals demanded and normally got what they considered to be the best equipment, assuming they had found sufficiently generous backers. Amateurs, however, were probably more inhibited in their approach for two reasons. Firstly few of the clubs could afford always to replace existing boats by those of a new kind and this inability to keep up with innovative design was one way in which clubs differed from each other, the larger metropolitan clubs having a decided advantage. Secondly, these new boats demanded considerable adaptation in the style of rowing and a good many amateurs found it hard to come to terms with what was needed. Woodgate, recalling his own years as an active oarsman during the 1860s, reckoned that it was rare to find an amateur at that time 'who could hit the time at scratch and could sit a rolling boat'. A rare exception, in his opinion, was Warre. E. D. Brickwood had no doubt that during the 1860s, coaches and oarsmen found it difficult to come to terms with the new type of boats in spite of their increase of pace: 'A great portion of the faulty style of today is to be attributed to the wholesale adoption of the modern racing boat, with all its difficulties', he wrote in 1866. The professionals, on the other hand, seem to have found few real problems in this way, perhaps because they had greater time for practice.[35] What was needed of all these oarsmen, if they were to cope, was a considerable degree of flexibility. At first, in the gig-type boats available, the stroke seems to have been of a short digging nature, probably with a marked lug at the finish. The shape of the boats and the manner in which the oarsmen were placed almost certainly dictated such a method. Each oarsman's feet would have been placed by the side of the oarsman in front of him and this would have restricted any marked swing towards the catch.[36] Modifications were probably made to boats of this kind but how far they allowed any degree of real swing is uncertain. Leander was reported as introducing 'a slow dwelling stroke', while Lehmann recorded that reaching out to the catch was already becoming common by the mid-1830s. Cambridge, he went on, adopted this approach earlier than Oxford, where it was not until 1841–2 that the combined efforts of Shadwell and Fletcher Menzies introduced a longer stroke.[37] Others, however, suggest otherwise. Woodgate remembered seeing the former Cambridge blue of the mid-1840s, F. M. Arnold, paddling on the river at a time when he was admittedly long past his prime. 'His style was interesting,' he wrote, 'very long, with a great heave into the chest at the finish and a long swing back, an emblem of the heavy-boat style, when a sharp catch at the beginning . . . was not so practicable.'[38] Whatever the truth of the matter, the elongation of the outrigged eight seems to have affected the manner in which they were rowed since such boats did not always run well between strokes. The answer seems to have been to concentrate on a high rating. The Oxford boat of 1852, coached by Menzies and the apostate Egan, was probably rowed in this particular way, one of its members, R. Greenall, being able to extract a rating of fifty out of his Brasenose crew when he took them to the headship of the river at Oxford that year.[39] Nor was such rapidity of stroke always abandoned after the slide was introduced. Dr Warre would not allow slides longer than eight to ten inches and occasionally his crews took undue advantage of these miniscule mechanisms. Bourne relates how, when he was at school, the Eton eight got in fifty-one strokes in a minute's row: 'Dr. Warre was furious and sent us back to row another minute at a much slower rate. This time we put in 49 strokes, and McCalmount could not be convinced that he had not carried out Dr. Warre's instructions to the letter.'[40]

In 1857 Oxford, in their Matthew Taylor-built boat, used Taylor as coach during part of their training to instruct them how to manage the new keelless eight. Cambridge had never totally abandoned such professional help and it may well be that, given the various changes that were taking place in the design of boats, they were wise. Exactly what the best amateurs were really doing remains confusing, especially as the business of coaching was still in its infancy.[41] Byrne and Churchill wondered whether the famous *cri de coeur* in 1852 of T. S. Egan might be interpreted as a demand for formalism that could easily lead some to sacrifice pace for dressage points, an ever-present danger in practically all styles and with every coach of whatever age or time.[42] But this does not seem to have been the case with the professionals, at least during the classic period of their dominance until the 1870s, when they managed to combine innovatory skills in boat-building and design with equally important experiments into the best ways of moving these new boats. *The Times* could report of Clasper's crew of 1844 that 'the Newcastle men had a stroke peculiar to themselves', while the highest tribute that A. A. Casamajor could pay to a member of the 1858 Oxford crew was to say that his method 'was founded exactly upon the Clasper style'.[43] It seems probable that that these professionals had discovered the need for length, a good catch and an accelerated stroke in order to move their light craft effectively and to stop the boat running away from them. *Bell's Life* wrote in August 1859 of Robert Chambers that his style was 'magnificent and few who saw him row that latter part of race will ever forget that majestic, even, and stupendous sweep of the sculls, or the finished fall of his compact shoulders, and his back of well defined muscles'.[44] It has perhaps been too readily assumed by some, G. C. Bourne among them, that there was some kind of natural progression from the early principles of Shadwell and Egan to those of Dr Warre and the full flowering of the orthodox style. In fact it may well be that the real importance of the first two lies in the part they played in creating a particular climate of opinion that, in its turn, allowed the full gospel of Dr Warre to flourish but that the latter's main debt, as far as rowing was concerned, was to the professionals. It was not without consequence that he rowed at six in the 1857 Oxford boat that had Matthew Taylor as one of its coaches.

The other major development, that of the sliding seat, was an American invention but the idea of moving on a fixed seat had become common enough among the Tyne professionals by the 1860s. J. H.

Clasper, Harry Clasper's son, slid for spurting purposes as early as 1857 and both Chambers and Renforth did the same.[45] W. Fawcus of Tynemouth RC used a similar tactic when winning the Diamonds and the Wingfields in 1871 and appears to have profited from the advice of the professionals with whom he shared the river, while J. H. Clasper induced the Cambridge blue, J. H. D. Goldie, to use olive oil on his seat when he was training for the Diamonds in the same year.[46] Others tried other methods. H. A. Freeman, a well-known amateur sculler on the Tideway of the same vintage, placed a sheet of plate glass on the seat of his sculling boat.[47] Tom Winship, another Tyne professional, had coached the John O'Gaunt four from Lancaster to slide when they were rowing in the Stewards at Henley in 1870 but they made the mistake of trying the method over the whole course and the effort, combined with the skin-friction, seems to have tired them out.[48] They would probably have done better to have followed the methods of the professionals and used the stratagem for spurts only. That apparently was the way Renforth's crew behaved in Canada when winning the World Championship there in 1870.[49]

Chambers, who apparently suffered some discomfort from his sliding tactics, more than once expressed the wish that someone would build a small bogie on wheels.[50] It remains odd, given the inventive skill of the Tyne oarsmen, that nobody followed up this suggestion. The only reference to an early moving seat in this country is to R. O. Birch who appears to have used one at King's Lynn Regatta during the summer of 1870.[51] On the other side of the Atlantic, however, J. C. Babcock had fitted a crude sliding seat to a sculling boat as early as 1857 but did not pursue the idea any further until 1869, when he fitted similar seats to a six-oared boat. They were ten-inch squares of wood, covered in leather and with grooves at the edges to slide on brass tracks.[52] Another American, Walter Brown, a professional sculler, had similarly experimented with a sliding mechanism in 1861 but took the invention no further.[53] In November 1869, Brown, at that time the American champion, rowed against the Thames oarsman, William Sadler, but it was decided to hold the match on the Tyne. Brown based himself at the Ord Arms Inn at Scotswood which was also being used at the same time as the headquarters of a Tyne four. One of its crew was James Taylor, brother of Matthew Taylor, and, in 1870, one of Renforth's four in Canada. Brown apparently observed the Tyne crew in training and saw their attempts at sliding. It seems inconceivable that between them they did not discuss the idea of his early moveable seat. The idea, therefore, was much in the air and it may have jogged Brown to reconsider his original seat when he returned to the United States. What seems clear is that when the Tyne men went to Canada in 1870 and 1871, they went with an open mind about the possibility of a moving seat and they may well have raced against crews, in practice, that were using crude versions of the mechanism.[54]

There had been two Tyne crews in Canada in 1871, arguments having led to a split in the original combination of the previous year. That which was captained by James Taylor deeply resented not being allowed itself to challenge for the championship and, on their return to the Tyne, arranged a match against the other four, a replacement being found for Renforth. Taylor's crew had shown considerable interest in the sliding seat while in Canada and, on arriving back on the Tyne, Taylor fitted up two sculling boats with experimental slides. Imperfect as these mechanisms probably were – early slides were normally bone runners in steel grooves – they were fitted to Taylor's new coxswainless four and his crew easily won the race. Both Thames RC and London RC took an immediate interest in this new development. F. S. Gulston of London had a slide fitted to his sculling boat in December 1871 and not long afterwards to a coxswainless four, inviting the professional, Joseph Sadler, who had been in the winning Tyne four, to join his crew in practice rows.[55] It was after these experiments that London RC decided to fit slides for the fours' race against the Atalanta Club of New York in May 1872 and their fairly easy victory led to considerable interest in their use. At the 1872 Henley all the London RC crews used them and Pembroke College, Cambridge, won the Visitors using wheeled slides. Thames RC, however, have some claim to being the first amateur club to use slides. According to W. H. Eyre, a tub-eight was fitted with them and used for practice during the winter of 1871–2 and, soon afterwards, Thames RC ordered a new eight with slides from Jewett of Dunston.[56]

Some prejudices remained, not least because it took some ten or more years to devise an appropriately sound type of sliding seat. They were not used in the Boat Race until 1873, although J. H. Clasper had tried to persuade Cambridge to use them the previous year.[57] Nor, after all the initial excitement, was it immediately obvious that they increased the pace of a boat. R. D. Burnell has drawn attention to the fact that, both at Henley and in the Boat Race, times actually slowed down following the introduction of the slide.[58] One obvious reason is that it took time for coaches and oarsmen to discover exactly how to exploit the new device. Bourne recalled how, as a boy at Eton, he had watched one of the Oxford crews of the early 1880s at practice. He wrote that

> the slide and swing were no longer in unison. The slide was held fast against the front-stop at the beginning of the stroke while the body was swung up to the perpendicular as if on a fixed seat, and then, and not till then, the slide was brought into use and the legs forcibly extended. The long swing back was a necessary result of delaying the use of the slide for so long.[59]

Rowe and Pitman thought that Cambridge, especially after slides were extended in length to 14 and 16 inches, were the first to come to terms with the problems presented by slides and they particularly instanced the combination of good sliding and powerful leg-work of the Cambridge crew in 1888.[60] As far as sculling was concerned, Woodgate gave special praise to the style of the American professional, Edward Hanlan, who held the sculling championship six times between 1879 and 1884, all his races except the last being on the Tyne or the Thames: 'Hanlan used his slide concurrently with swing, carrying his body well back, with straight arms long past the perpendicular, before he attempted to row the stroke in by bending the arms.'[61] He argued that the best of the English professionals of an earlier generation would have adapted just as well and he recalled seeing Harry Kelley, long since retired, trying out a sculling boat with a sliding seat: 'His style was a model for all our young school to copy', he claimed, condemning at the same time most of the scullers he had seen with the exception of Frank Playford and T. C. Edwards-Moss.[62]

A further handicap, however, may well have been the standard of the oars in use at the time. Unfortunately far less is known about their development than almost any other piece of equipment. The earliest ones were heavy, square-loomed affairs, often weighted down with lead at the handle, the blades being long and straight. Scooped blades had made their appearance on the Thames by the early 1840s and were used by Coombes's crew in his defeat of the Clasper four in 1842. Nor, given the shape of the boats, were all the oars of a similar length, Taylor's eight for Royal Chester probably being the first craft constructed for oars that were exactly similar.[63] Harry Clasper made some experiments, using both scooped blades and round looms, and what became known as the Newcastle oar was in reasonably common use by the 1850s.[64] Not all Clasper's attempts were successful. He was beaten in a coxed pair match in August 1847, *The Times* commenting that Clasper's style differed markedly from his previous efforts. In this particular case, apparently, he was using an oar shorter than normal and, in doing so, he was raising an issue that was to cause considerable argument up to 1914 about what exactly the suitable length of an oar should be and what should be the inboard to outboard ratio.[65]

During the 1880s, various different shapes of blades emerged. Dr Warre used coffin oars at one time with his Eton crews, the widest point being some ten inches from the tip. Others preferred barrel shaped blades where the broadest part was 6 to 8 inches from the end to the more normal square blade with the widest part at the tip.[66] But the most important developments were those that strengthened the oar so that they could more effectively be used with the sliding seat. The crucial point came with the 1887 Boat Race. D. H. McLean, rowing seven in the Oxford crew, broke his oar clean off just after Barnes Bridge, probably through hitting a wave on the way forward. The weakness was caused by the leather being nailed to the loom and Ayling's, the oar makers, immediately patented a means of keeping it in place by means of a brass plate.[67] Stiffening the oars, however, to prevent twisting was a more difficult problem to solve. Bourne still had a preference for solid oars during the mid-1920s, although he accepted that the tubular variety, first used in this country by the Belgians before the Great War, were superior in stiffness.[68] A variation of the solid oar was the girder construction, with one or two grooves on either side of the loom. These were considered by both Bourne and Lehmann, who introduced them from America in 1897, as the best available but only if made with properly seasoned wood.[69]

By the 1870s and 1880s the modern racing boat had essentially arrived, not greatly different in shape from those in use today but almost always made of wood. In America, papier-mâché was occasionally used for a boat's skin and Columbia brought such a craft to Henley in 1878 but decided in the end to race in a wooden one.[70] The majority of boats before 1914 remained side-seated, an arrangement that was supposed to assist balance but centre-seated craft were beginning to emerge during the 1880s, Eton using such a boat under Dr Warre, always something of an innovator.[71] Encouraging the continued use of side-seated boats was the general weakness of the riggers. Experiments at Cambridge in 1891, largely following the introduction of improved bicycle construction, led to Caius College fitting tubular steel outriggers to their eight and, once Matthew Wood of Putney began to produce them after 1896, they were rapidly accepted, being both lighter and stronger.[72] The swivel rowlock was introduced from the United States during the late 1870s. Although quickly adopted for sculling boats, the oarsmen and coaches remained divided until the Second World War about their merits. The universities and colleges were the more conservative but elsewhere, especially on the metropolitan Thames, they gained more favour.[73] Equally contrary opinions were expressed about cambered boats. The first ever seen in this country was the cigar-shaped sculling boat brought by the Australian professional, R. A. W. Green, in 1863, although he quickly abandoned its use once he had experienced the contrary waters of the Tideway. James Taylor subsequently developed a cambered sculling boat in 1870 on the Tyne but, whenever such boats were used, they proved difficult to steer in a strong wind. Various devices were used to counteract this, including a small wind-sail on the bow, but it was not until J. H. Clasper invented and patented a fin-keel that the problem was resolved.[74] There were some, including Woodgate, who regarded the use of a fin as the equivalent of questioning an oarsman's manhood. He viewed them with distaste and, except in a side-wind, as an 'actual encumbrance'.[75]

The changes in design and shape of boats inevitably meant adjustments and alterations to the style of rowing. Because the stakes were often high, the matches of the professionals gave them sufficient encouragement to experiment with different methods. The occasional amateur, such as Woodgate, may in his youth have inspired change, more particularly the adoption among amateurs of the coxswainless four, and Dr Warre at Eton was fertile with new ideas. But for the most part, they remained a conservative group, prepared to accept innovations only after they had been proven by the professionals. The final achievements of the latter, often rough-hewn men, were things of beauty, the lines of which have withstood the test of time. Not the least noteworthy part of their craftsmanship was their rejection of conjecture and theory in favour of experience and practical experiment. They tested their boats against each other relentlessly, in particular during the often fierce struggles between the Tyne and the Thames. In terms of inventiveness the Tyne always had the edge and the tradition of good boat-building continued on that river until the eve of the Great War.

Notes

1 L. S. R. Byrne and E. L. Churchill, *The Eton Book of the River* (Eton, 1935), pp. 236–7.
2 *Ibid.*, p. 242; *The Times*, 24 July 1871.
3 G. C. Drinkwater and T. R. B. Saunders, *The University Boat Race, 1829–1929* (London, 1929), p. 175.
4 Byrne and Churchill, *The Eton Book*, p. 242.

5 Stonehenge, *British Rural Sports* (London, 1861), p. 472.
6 W. B. Woodgate, *Boating* (London, 1888), p. 142; Drinkwater and Saunders, *Boat Race*, p. 205.
7 T. A. Cook and Guy Nickalls, *Thomas Doggett Deceased* (London, 1908), p. 68.
8 W. E. Sherwood, *Oxford Rowing* (Oxford and London, 1900), p. 11; *The Field*, 20 December 1913.
9 A. A. Macfarlane-Grieve, *A History of Durham Rowing* (Newcastle, 1922), p. 23; Argonaut, (E. D. Brickwood), *The Arts of Rowing and Training* (London, 1866), p. 5.
10 Argonaut, *The Arts*, p. 5.
11 R. P. P. Rowe and C. M. Pitman, *Rowing* (London, 1898), p. 15.
12 Byrne and Churchill, *The Eton Book*, pp. 243–4; *Newcastle Daily Chronicle*, 1 July 1861, 13 March 1909.
13 *Tyne Mercury*, 19 July 1842.
14 *Ibid.*, 25 June 1844; *The British Rowing Almanack*, 1863, p. 98.
15 W. B. Woodgate, *Boating* (London, 1888), p. 301.
16 *Newcastle Journal*, 14, 21 December 1944; T. A. Cook, *Rowing at Henley* (London, 1919), p. 95.
17 *Newcastle Journal*, 28 December 1844.
18 Christopher Dodd, *Henley Royal Regatta* (London, 1981), p. 56.
19 Argonaut, *The Arts*, p. 7.
20 *Newcastle Daily Chronicle*, 13, 20 March 1909.
21 Cook, *Rowing*, p. 79.
·22 *Ibid.*, p. 80; *Newcastle Journal*, 24 May, 1845.
23 R. D. Burnell, *Henley Regatta – A History* (London, 1957), pp. 76–7.
24 Drinkwater and Saunders, *Boat Race*, p. 175.
25 *Newcastle Journal*, 22 March 1845; *Illustrated London News*, 29 March 1845.
26 Woodgate, *Boating*, p. 175; Drinkwater and Saunders, *Boat race*. p. 175; R. C. Lehmann, *Rowing* (London, 1898), pp. 8–9; *The Complete Oarsman* (London, 1908), p. 21.
27 R. D. Burnell, *Swing Together* (London, 1952), pp. 8–9; Cook, *Rowing*, p. 81.
28 *Illustrated London News*, 29 March 1845.
29 Cook, *Rowing*, p. 105; G. C. Bourne, *A Text-Book of Oarsmanship* (London, 1925), p. 206.
30 Burnell, *Henley Regatta*, p. 86.
31 *The Field*, 16 March 1901.
32 Bourne, *Text-Book*, pp. 203–4.
33 Cook, *Rowing*, pp. 82–3; Drinkwater and Saunders, *Boat Race*, p. 178; Byrne and Churchill, *The Eton Book*, pp. 246–7.
34 Cook, *Boat Race*, p. 84.
35 W. B. Woodgate in *The Sportsman, British Sports and Sportsmen* (London, 1916), pp. 366–8; Argonaut, *The Arts*, p. 8.
36 Byrne and Churchill, *The Eton Book*, p. 200; Burnell, *Swing Together*, p. 8.
37 Byrne and Churchill, *ibid.*; Lehmann, *Complete Oarsman*, pp. 26–8.
38 Woodgate in *British Sports*, p. 341.
39 *The Field*, 16 March 1901.
40 G. C. Bourne, *Memories of an Eton Wet-Bob of the Seventies* (London, 1933), p. 97; R. J. Elles, 'The short-slide controversy', *Cambridge Review*, 2 November 1928.

41 Woodgate in *British Sports*, p. 362.
42 Byrne and Churchill, *The Eton Book*, p. 246.
43 *The Times*, 24 June 1844; Lehmann, *Complete Oarsman*, p. 28.
44 *Bell's Sporting Life in London*, 21 August 1859; Argonaut, *The Arts*, p. 78 where Brickwood comments on Chambers' 'marvellous length combined with effectiveness.'
45 *Newcastle Daily Chronicle*, 3 April 1909; *The Field*, 15 January, 26 February, 23 April, 1910.
46 *The Field*, 26 February 1910.
47 *Ibid.*
48 Woodgate, *Boating*, p. 104.
49 *Ibid.*
50 *The Field*, 26 February, 23 April, 1910.
51 Woodgate, *Boating*, p. 104.
52 *Ibid.*, pp. 105; Byrne and Churchill, *The Eton Book*, pp. 247–8; Burnell, *Swing Together*, p. 9.
53 Woodgate, *Boating*, p. 106.
54 *Newcastle Daily Chronicle*, 3 April 1909; *The Field*, 26 February 1910; Woodgate, *Rowing*, p. 105.
55 Woodgate, *Rowing*, p. 105; *The Field*, 12 March 1910.
56 *The Field*, 19, 26 February 1910; Woodgate, *Rowing*, pp. 105–6; Burnell, *Swing Together*, p. 9.
57 Drinkwater and Saunders, *Boat Race*, pp. 65–6.
58 Burnell, *Swing Together*, pp. 17–9.
59 Bourne, *Eton Wet-Bob*, pp. 90–1.
60 Rowe and Pitman, *Rowing*, pp. 55–6.
61 Woodgate, *Rowing*, p. 227.
62 *Ibid.*, pp. 227–8; Rowe and Pitman, *Rowing*, pp. 52–3.
63 Byrne and Churchill, *The Eton Book*, pp. 238, 246; Lehmann, *Complete Oarsman*, p. 23; *Newcastle Journal*, 13 July 1870.
64 Byrne and Churchill, *The Eton Book*, p. 239; *The Field*, 7 April 1900.
65 *The Times*, 11 August 1847; *The Field*, 29 April 1911; Bourne, *Text-Book*, pp. 167–92; Cook, *Rowing*, pp. 65–72; Lehmann, *Complete Oarsman*, pp. 69–70.
66 Lehmann, *Complete Oarsman*, p. 70; Bourne, *Text-Book*, p. 184.
67 Drinkwater and Saunders, *Boat Race*, pp. 90–1.
68 Bourne, *Text-Book*, p. 190.
69 *Ibid*; Lehmann, *Complete Oarsman*, p. 23; Byrne and Churchill, *The Eton Book*, pp. 251–2; E. McGruer, 'Notes on oar building', *Cambridge Magazine*, 3 May 1919.
70 Christopher Dodd, *Henley*, p. 66.
71 Lehmann, *Complete Oarsman*, p. 69; Bourne, *Text-Book*, p. 215; Bourne, *Wet-Bob*, p. 65; Cook, *Rowing*, pp. 91–2.
72 Byrne and Churchill, *The Eton Book*, p. 252.
73 *The Field*, 18 June 1908.
74 *Bell's Life*, 16 June 1863; *Newcastle Daily Chronicle*, 21 March 1870, 20 March 1909.
75 Woodgate in *British Sports*, p. 362.

Appendix II – Health and training

Writing in 1884, Dr Warre rejoiced at the abandonment of the training methods of an earlier age. He attributed most of the faults of the older approach to too great a dependence on the views and practices of the professionals. In particular, he correctly picked out the dietary defects of the former generation – any amount of meat as long as it was under-done, stale bread, hardly any vegetables and severe restrictions on the amount an oarsman should be allowed to drink. Warre also based his criticisms of what he believed to be the professionals' approach, on the interesting social argument that, as a rule, men of that kind would from necessity accept an inferior standard of food and drink. Only before an important race was a waterman likely to be properly fed and watered: 'His training, to get into condition if he was backed for a race, was a period of unusual luxury for him.'[1] By implication, therefore, the regime that they recommended was hardly relevant to members of the praetorian guard.

Warre's direct experience of the dietary habits of the average wherry-man, lighterman or miner must have been slight. He may perhaps have been unduly influenced by the prejudices of the only professional he had come to know well, Matthew Taylor, coach for a time of the 1857 Oxford crew. He certainly long remembered Taylor's total dislike of the idea of an oarsman having a bath after an outing.[2] There seems no doubt that some of the misunderstanding about these early professional coaches was based on too great an acceptance of some of their whims. Shadwell warned against these as early as 1846:

> We will only say that under the name of training there is often much extravagance practised, enveloped in a proportionate degree of mystery, as is especially the case where watermen are employed, under the influence of which the rowing men became exceedingly scrupulous about insignificant

trifles, and look upon that part of the training as the one grand thing they have to care for.[3]

Nevertheless there remained some idiosyncratic and even dangerous precepts, largely based on ignorance, of which the most prevalent was the worry about internal fat. Shadwell was one who was alarmed about this. Although he advanced the sensible enough notion that 'the only really necessary things to be adhered to are moderation in eating, drinking and sleeping', he warned against 'internal fat, which most people in health have, and which is the great enemy of good wind . . . But all will be of no use unless the liquors are cut off, for it is through them that the internal fat is produced, and especially by beer.'[4] Archibald Maclaren, who ran a gymnasium in Oxford and had some experience of rowing, was to indicate the error of this kind of thinking in an important book published in 1866. He recognised, however, that many of these ideas were firmly rooted and that it might take time to dispel them. It was not going to be easy to dissuade those who, as he put it, believed perspiration to be 'only fat in a state of melt'.[5]

The danger of a limited and restricted diet, especially the rationing of liquids, is underlined by the kind of work on the water that the best crews were doing. The regime demanded of the 1858 Cambridge crew is typical. Work on sorting out the best oarsmen had begun in the Michaelmas Term 1857 and continued for some weeks after the New Year. By 24 February the eight had been chosen and, apart from some rearrangement in its order and the occasional substitute because of illness, was the crew that defeated Oxford on 27 March. Egan was asked to look after the coaching while Shadwell was in charge at Oxford. Egan had four and a half weeks to get the crew into shape in what turned out to be singularly inhospitable weather. Running a mile or so was demanded before breakfast and occasionally after an outing. There were six outings each week, all of them consisting of long rows at a low rating to Baitsbyke, Clayhithe or Bottisham, plus the occasional paddle to Ely and back which took two days. There was nothing particularly odd about this schedule apart from its drudgery. But it sounds as if Egan was indulging in a form of steady-state with men, most of whom would have been reasonably fit following the various trials and the demands of collegiate rowing. What was surprising was what followed. During its last week on the Cam, the crew rowed a lock to lock each day. The times were 21 minutes 55 seconds, 20 minutes 40 seconds, 21 minutes 08 seconds, 20 minutes 46 seconds, 21 minutes 07 seconds and 20 minutes

28 seconds, the last being the fastest recorded to that date. It took Cambridge two days to get themselves and their new Matthew Taylor boat to Putney and then they proceeded to row three full courses from Mortlake to Putney over successive days, one of them against a scratch eight of watermen whom they beat after giving them a two length start. Only on the Friday was there any diminution of effort, the crew being content with a row of just over eight minutes. In the ten outings prior to the Boat Race, the Cambridge crew had done just over 200 minutes of full-pressure work with no apparent rest other than the two days that it took them to get to the Thames. By any standard it was a punishing enough programme. Not the least of its oddities was that never once did the crew appear to practise in the actual direction of the race, all the main pieces being on the ebb. Oxford, arriving three days earlier on the Tideway, managed four full courses and would have done more had it not been for illness and damage to their boat. At least they took the precaution of rowing one of these trials on the flood.[6]

Apparently, if Maclaren is to be believed, such feats of endurance were becoming the object of adverse comment among a widening circle of interested and alarmed onlookers.[7] F. C. Skey, a surgeon and a Fellow of the Royal Society, was the first to articulate these fears in a letter to *The Times* in October 1867. He felt 'that there is no more palpable example of cruelty than consists of putting against each other two or more antagonists with a view to determine whose physical prowess are capable of most endurance . . . and of this form of cruelty to animals no modern example is so great as the annual University Boat Race'. He argued that 'the price is exorbitant' and 'that the University Boat Race as at present established is a national folly'.[8] *The Times*, while recognising the worries of the likes of Skey, pointed out that there was no hard and fast evidence on which to make a proper judgement.[9] In 1873 this was supplied in *University Oars*, written by J. E. Morgan, a Manchester consultant and former oarsman, who with great assiduity corresponded with all living rowing blues from 1829 to 1869 and with the families of those who had died.

It remains an odd book. As might be expected from a medical man, Morgan wrote with some care and a good deal of sense about the stresses and strains on the human body under extreme physical exertion. He properly gave the advice that if 'training be commenced gradually and carried out systematically, it will be the means of strengthening the muscles of the heart and the vascular system'.[10] But, as far as his main enquiry was concerned, he basically got the answers that he wanted.

Only seventeen of the 294 oarsmen with whom he corresponded admitted to any long-term injury as a result of their rowing.[11] The great majority considered that rowing had benefited them and that their good health was a direct result of their activities on the river. But tucked away in the volume were a number who voiced doubts and worries. One was Charles Wordsworth, largely responsible for the first race in 1829. 'There is a limit,' he wrote, 'beyond which the practice of rowing, especially in races, cannot be carried without injury, more or less serious both to body and mind, and I sadly fear that this limit may have been exceeded at the present day.'[12] Another, H. A. Morgan, Fellow and Tutor of Jesus College, Cambridge, where he was in fact an enthusiastic supporter of the college boat club, confessed nevertheless that he had on occasions 'noticed a certain worn-out expression about former university oarsmen. Without being ill, they appear to be fit for little active exertion.'[13]

In fact Morgan's book was published at a time when there were already considerable changes in training methods. The two editions of Maclaren's book are witness to that and they may well have been an important contribution to modifying some of the earlier excesses. In the preface to the second edition he claimed to detect a new approach to training:

> Altogether a more rational and common-sense view of the subject is being gradually entertained . . . The mischievous habit of amateur physicking is being abandoned, and the dangerous custom of forced perspirations, undertaken to exorcise the demon of 'internal fat' and 'loose flesh' may be said to be discarded.[14]

In this edition, Maclaren extended the arguments of his 1866 book above all by continually emphasising the principle of gradual and progressive preparation as the essence of training and by combining this with a common sense approach to eating and drinking.[15] Nevertheless, important as Maclaren's two volumes were, it was to take time before all the ancient prejudices were dispelled. Woodgate, writing in 1888, although advocating an entirely sensible approach to training on the water, still showed some reluctance about abandoning the restrictions on drinking.[16] Ten years later, however, R. P. P. Rowe and C. M. Pitman were totally converted: 'In many clubs the ridiculous practice still survives of limiting the whole crew, large and small, fat and thin, to so many pints of liquid a day. There can be no greater error than to allow a man too little to drink.'[17]

By the end of the century, methods of training were better considered and applied. Coaches and oarsmen were certainly well informed compared with those of only the recent past. It may be that they did less work than in former times but it was qualitatively better than had once been the case. Alarm, however, still continued to be expressed about the effects of rowing on a man's health. R. C. Lehmann was forced to defend the sport from charges brought against it in the *St James' Gazette* in 1898. He was particuarly concerned because of the implication that the deaths of three recent Oxford oarsmen – H. B. Cotton, T. H. E Stretch and E. R. Balfour – were directly due to their rowing. Stretch was the victim of a burst appendix at a time when the operation for that problem was only in its infancy. Lehmann persuaded himself that the deaths of the other two – Cotton's influenza leading to pneumonia and then consumption and Balfour's chill to congested lungs and kidney failure – had nothing to do with rowing. In the light of modern knowledge of the potential danger of taking exercises while suffering from a virus complaint, his defence was perhaps less than reassuring. But, fair-minded as Lehmann was, he did admit the foolishness of claiming 'that rowing confers an immunity from fatal illness'. What was more interesting was his total rejection of the suggestion that there were other ways of training an oarsman, for example, by using exercises in a gymnasium, a possibility that Maclaren had thought was worth exploring. Lehmann concluded that:

> the method of training and development that may fit a man admirably for the purpose of weight-lifting, or of excelling his fellow-creatures in the measurement of his chest and his muscles, is utterly unsuited for a contest that requires great quickness of movement, highly developed lung-power, and general endurance spread over a period of some twenty minutes.[18]

It was an argument that was to continue for many years to come.

Training for any athletic pursuit was, during the 1840s and the 1850s, in a rudimentary state. It seems more than probable that men at that time knew far more about how to bring a horse up to racing pitch than how to cope with the human body under any form of stress. A great deal was based on myth and ignorance and only time and more certain knowledge could lead to a more rational system. It seems a pity that the likes of Dr Warre and others could put much of the blame for some of the early faults and errors on the shoulders of the professionals. The fierce demands placed on the Boat Race crews of 1858 were the consequence of using Shadwell and Egan as coaches, not of employing watermen. Harry Clasper's own system of training for an important match seems not unreasonable compared with that imposed on the university oarsmen. He recommended four or five hours walking or rowing a day, divided between the morning and the afternoon with eight or nine hours sleep a night. He described his diet as limited but it still included chops for breakfast and beef or mutton at the midday meal. Vegetables were ignored but in that Clasper merely echoed the prejudices of his time. As for liquids, he allowed himself tea at breakfast, a glass of ale and one of port at 12.00 noon, doubling the amount of beer if no port was available. He drank more tea after the second outing and contented himself with a form of gruel in the evening. It was not an unreasonable approach to an active rowing life.[19] Nor were these men fools and their comments could on occasions reveal a wry and ironic view of some of the amateurs placed under their charge. Robert Coombes, Clasper's great rival and a coach of Cambridge during the 1840s and the early 1850s, wrote of the man who

> may be a fine oar and have pulled in the University Boat Race before, but that ought not to make him despise training when he is again elected . . . I remember Mr. ——, who had won everything before him, being in very bad training when he rowed a second time in the University crew. I always told him so; and yet he could speak and shout in the middle of a hard trial, when all the rest were done to a whisper. Why, a man who does this dispirits the others.[20]

Plus ça change, plus c'est la même chose.

Notes

1 E. Warre, 'Athletics: or physical exercise and recreation', Pt. I, X, General Hygiene, *The Health Exhibition Literature* (London, 1884), pp. 86–7.
2 *Ibid.*, pp. 89–90.
3 Anonymous (A. T. W. Shadwell), *Principles of Rowing* (London, 1846), p. 16.
4 *Ibid.*, p. 17.
5 Archibald Maclaren, *Training in Theory and Practice* (London, first ed. 1866), pp. 31–2.
6 A full account of the 1858 Cambridge crew and its training can be found in W. F. Macmichael, *The Oxford and Cambridge Boat Races* (Cambridge, 1870), pp. 238–251 and G. G. T. Treherne and J. H. D. Goldie, *Record of the University Boat Race 1829–1833* (London, 1884), pp. 83–7.
7 Archibald Maclaren, *Training in Theory and Practice* (London, second ed., 1874), p. 165.
8 *The Times*, 10 October 1867.
9 *Ibid.*, 15 October 1867.
10 J. E. Morgan, *University Oars, Being A Critical Enquiry into the After Health of the Men who Rowed in the Oxford and Cambridge Boat Race, 1829–1869* (London, 1873), p. 61.
11 *Ibid.*, Table IV, p. 378.
12 *Ibid.*, pp. 300–1.
13 *Ibid.*, p. 338.
14 Maclaren, (second ed.), pp. v–vi.

15 *Ibid.*, Pt. IV, 'A practical course of training', *passim.*
16 W. B. Woodgate, *Boating* (London, 1888), pp. 161–3.
17 R. P. P. Rowe and C. M. Pitman, *Rowing* (London, 1898), p. 106.
18 R. C. Lehmann, *Rowing* (London, 1898), pp. 288–306.
19 Maclaren, (second ed.), p. 226.
20 Robert Coombes, 'Hints on rowing and training in a member of the CUBC', *Aquatic Notes* (Cambridge, 1852), pp. 101–7.

Appendix III – The North-East music-halls and the Tyne professionals

A great many strands in public entertainment led to the Victorian music-hall. Some, such as the London pleasure gardens, dated back to the eighteenth century, the best known, the Vauxhall, not closing until 1859.[1] By the 1840s singing saloons were beginning to appear, often built by enterprising publicans as extensions to public houses.[2] Purpose-built music-halls began to appear throughout the country from the 1850s onwards and by 1866 outnumbered straight theatres by some five or six to one.[3] Ornate and often splendid buildings, some of them capable of holding 2,000 people, they attracted all sorts and conditions of men and women, but they were particularly important as places of working-class entertainment. The audiences, often braced with drink, demanded from the performers considerable skill and virtuosity. Those who passed muster could become popular household names, a significant element in the working-class culture of the day.

Like the rest of the country, the North East shared in this form of entertainment, Balmbra's Music Hall at Newcastle being especially well-known. The growth of the music-hall in the region coincided with the years when the Tyne professional oarsmen were at their majestic best. There was no particular stock-in-trade for those who performed on these stages. Humour and pathos were mixed together in song and dialogue over a whole range of subjects, from the trivial domestic situation to important national events. But the peculiar and distinct dialect of the north-eastern region, particularly the Geordie accent of Tyneside, placed a special onus on the performer to reflect events that had happened locally. One theme that audiences came to expect was some form of immediate comment on the triumphs and the tragedies of the professional oarsmen of the day, particularly Harry Clasper, Robert Chambers and James Renforth. Three entertainers, each in his way of considerable merit, coincided with the most famous years of these oarsmen. For Edward (Ned) Corvan (1829–65), George Ridley (1835–64) and Joe Wilson (1841–75), the often titanic clashes between the Tyne oarsmen and those of the Thames provided material that immediately gained the applause and the sympathy of a north-eastern audience which saw these matches in terms that were unique in the history of rowing. Some fifty or so of their songs, together with others by less well-known or anonymous performers, have recently been traced and many of them are in the process of being collected and published by Keith Gregson.[4]

The earliest known song about rowing dates from the mid-1840s, just at the time when the first professionals were beginning to make their mark.[5] But it was the extraordinary achievements of the Tyne oarsmen during the next two decades or so that inspired the writing of most of those that have survived. The affinity between the two kinds of performance was a close one. Whether on the water or on the stage, they all had similar origins and faced adoring but critical and, occasionally, fickle audiences. They knew each other reasonably well and it was appropriate that Ridley should have given the first rendering of his most famous song, 'The Blaydon Races', at Harry Clasper's testimonial at Balmbra's on 5 June 1862.[6] Joe Wilson produced the largest number of rowing songs, some twenty or so, and appears to have had a particularly close relationship with the Tyne oarsmen, about whom, according to Gregson, he produced the consistently best songs.[7]

Corvan, on the other hand, wrote far fewer but the dramatic quality of those that have survived remains striking, in at least one instance producing a song that seems to better that of Wilson. Both wrote about the match on the Tyne on 19 April 1859 between the young Robert Chambers and Thomas White of Bermondsey. It was to prove an important race since, according to *Bell's Life*, 'it was this victory, in a measure unexpected, which was the principal cause of his being backed against Kelley'.[8] That challenge took place on the Thames the following September and Chambers became the first Tyne oarsman to take the Championship of England. It was the manner in which Corvan seemed to sense, more so than Wilson, the important consequence of Chambers' victory over White that lends his own song its quality.

This particular match in April 1859 had not been without its problems. White had immediately taken a slender lead which he then increased considerably when Chambers fouled a barge at the side of the river. It looked momentarily as if the race was over. But Chambers, showing for the first time that measured power which made him such a formidable opponent, slowly overhauled his rival, there almost being a foul between them in the process. By Scotswood Bridge, Chambers was well clear and won the race by five lengths.[9] Such were the bare bones of what happened.

Wilson began his song by setting the scene before the race had begun:

> As aw was gan alang the Close last Tuesday afternoon,
> Aw saw a lot o' bettin men towards the Jard Group run.
> Says aw tiv a fishwife stanin near, 'What's thor gan ti take place?'
> She stares at me and cries 'ye feul, why tis the greet boat race.'

He continues in this vein with a verse about a drunk making his way to the race and another about some bantering between 'sum cockney fellows' and 'a well knawn ruff'. He admits that for many of the spectators there was not much to see – 'Tho' we, like iverybody else got just a passin glance' – and then concludes with a description of the race:

> Mis awful shouts onward they flew just like the leetnin's flash.
> In the water they myede a dashin cut, so of course they cut a dash.
> An awd wife oot a public hoose, roared out frae off the hills,
> 'Gan on Bob, ma canny lad!' for she knew he liked her gills.
>
> Chambers put in all his strength about the Meadow's hoose,
> Twas then the Cockney began ti feel his efforts war ne use.,
> So he thowt he'd try (alt o it's not in any rowing rule)
> Ti myeke a FOUL o' Bob – he tried – but myede hissel THE FOOL.
>
> Byeth the men luiked very RED, tho they stripped ti the BUFF;
> The race was ower, Chambers had wun, and geen Tom White the huff,
> For TYNESIDE PLUCK had gained the day, an noo it is wor pride
> Ti say we can defy the world wive a CHAMPION frae Tyneside.

Wilson no doubt delighted his audience at the start of his song with the suggestion that there could have been anyone along the Tyne that day without any idea of what was going on. Corvan began his effort differently, simply producing a verse 'in praise o' honest Chambers, or Tyneside men, the pride'. That no doubt too would be greeted with rapturous applause and agreement. He then went straight into his account of the race, making the incident of fouling the barge central to his theme, suggesting, rightly or wrongly, that Chambers's poor steering was the result of fouling tactics on White's part:

> Stroke for stroke contendin', they sweep on wi the tide,
> Fortune seems impendin' the victor ti decide:
> At last the Cockney lossin' strength, the fowlin' game did steal,
> He leaves his watter ivery length, an runs Chambers iv a keel.
> *Spoken*: What a hulla baloo! Hoo the Cockney speeled away, ivery yen thowt

the race was over. Some said it was a deed robbery, others a worry, an wawk hyem before the finish o' the race. There was a chep stannin' aside me wiv his hands iv his pockets – aw'm sartin there wis nowt else in – liukin' on the river wiv a feyce like a fiddle-stick. He sung the followin' lament, efter the or 'There's nae Luck aboot the Hoose.'

Says one poor soul aw've selled my pigs, my clock, my drawers, an bed
An doon te Wawker a' mun wawk, then aw might a rode i'steed;
Gox! there's wor Jim an a' the crew's pawned ivery stitch o'claes,
And they say thor's two cheps selled their wives, the six ti fower te raise.

Chorus –
For oh! dismay upon that day in ornist did begin,
On ivry face a chep might trace – (Spoken) – who's forst, Bob? –
(Sings) – Oh! the Cockney's sure te win.

Ten lengths aheed – farewell bedsteed – maw achin beyns nae mair
On thou mun rowl, no! this poor soul mun rest on deep despair;
Wor Nannie, tee, she'll curse en flee, and belt me like a Tork,
For aw've lost my money, time, an spree, and mebies loss maw work.

The cleverness of the Corvan song and dialogue lies in the way he virtually ignores the actual race after the incident with the barge and instead concentrates all his efforts on the attitudes of the spectators, at one moment so full of hope and excitement, at the next reduced to alarm and anxiety at the possible consequences of White's foulings tactics. Even though the audience knew the final outcome, they must have been on edge at the implications of what Corvan was relating, no doubt many having experienced such bitter consequences at some time in the past. Relentlessly, he pushed this theme almost to the very end of the performance:

Spoken: Comin' doon after awe wis ower, aw meets one i' wor cheps, (an Irishman), they cawed him Patrick, but a call'd him Mick, for shortness. He waden't wait for the finish, altho' he backed Bob. So ah hailed him, 'Hie Mick, wo's forst?' – 'Go to blazes!' says he – 'Nonsense, Mick, who's forst?' – 'Och, shure,' says he, 'the Londin man was forst half-way before the race wis qarther over' – 'Had on, Mick, that's a Bull; did ye lay owt on tiv him, aw mean Bob?' – 'By my soul, I did! an I'd like to lay this lump ov a stick on his dirty conco-nut. The next time may I be struck wid a button on my upper lip as big as a clock face!' – 'But Chambers is forst,' says aw – 'Arrah? D'ye mane to say that?' say he – 'Didn't aw tel ye he'd win afore iver he started.' – Hurro! – More Power! – Fire Away!

Chorus: Singing' pull away, pull away, pull away, boys!
Pull away, boys, se clever,
Pull away, pull away, pull away, boys,
Chambers for iver![10]

222

Corvan's song and performance are instructive not just as an intelligent piece of music-hall skill – indicating that what must have seemed spontaneous was, in fact, the fruit of much thought about the reaction of his audience – for he goes further than that. Without denigrating Chambers's place in the folklore of Tyneside – and it should be remembered that at the time Chambers was still just a good local oarsman – Corvan manages to convey the complex attitudes of the crowd, not being afraid to remind his audience that many of them had been cruel and angry when they thought that White was going to win. He manages to bring out all the tensions that both inspired and ultimately drove those Tyne champions beyond the reasonable bounds of competition. In time, with so many victories behind him, Chambers could still retain the sympathy of his once inconstant followers even when he was defeated. Joe Wilson recognised this change in attitude when, in May 1867, Kelley defeated Chambers and deprived him of the championship. Wilson may well have known, as may possibly his audience, that Chambers was already weakened by the illness that was to lead to his death and that public demand was forcing the once great sculler to attempt something of which he was no longer capable: 'Tho lick't,' sang Wilson, 'yor still wor pride.'

These songs and performances were essentially parochial affairs, confined to the North East and more particularly to Tyneside. The Great Thames professionals do not seem to have inspired similar reactions in London. Possibly they had no need for such public praise since they saw themselves as the natural champions. The Tyneside men on the other hand, even when they were victorious, remained the challengers, constantly striving to usurp a position that the Thames men saw as theirs by right. They were fortunate to have men gifted in a different way who could chronicle their triumphs and as well as their disasters. The Tyneside crowd needed its heroes and in Clasper, Chambers and Renforth they found men who were out of the ordinary. It must remain, however, a matter of speculation how far the likes of Corvan, Ridley and Wilson encouraged still further the view that these oarsmen were so much the best in the field that in the end they overreached themselves. It would be pleasant to think that it was not the case. It would be more charitable to remember the coincidence of two different kinds of public performers who, together, created for some forty or so years a climate of excitement and admiration in what was a unique and idiosyncratic part of the kingdom.

Appendix III

Notes

1 Geoffrey Best, *Mid Victorian Britain 1851–75* (London, 1971), pp. 212–7.
2 F. M. L. Thompson, *The Rise of Respectable Society, A social History of Victorian Britain, 1830–1900* (London, 1988), p. 323.
3 Michael Baker. *The Rise of the Victorian Actor* (London, 1978), p. 127.
4 K. Gregson, 'When the boat came in – the songs of nineteenth-century sport', *English Dance and Song*, Winter, 1978; 'Bob Chambers: a much sung hero', *Newcastle Journal*, 27 June 1981; 'Songs of Tyneside boat racing', *North East Labour History*, no. 16, 1982; 'Champions at Talkin Tarn', *Cumbria Magazine*, *32, no. 6, 1982; Corvan – A Victorian Entertainer and His Songs*, (Banbury, 1983).
5 Gregson, *North East Labour History*, 1982.
6 *Newcastle Daily Chronicle*, 6 June 1862.
7 Gregson, *Corvan*, p. 6; *North East Labour History*, 1982.
8 *Bell's Life*, 20 September 1859.
9 *The Times*, 20 April 1859.
10 The two songs by Wilson and Corvan are to be found in Gregson, *North East Labour History, Corvan*, pp. 6–31.

Select bibliography

Minutes and printed documents (ARA headquarters, London)

Amateur Rowing Association – *Minutes*, 1934–60.
ARA Provincial Committee – *Minutes*, 1946–57.
Annual General Meetings, ARA Provincial Committee – Printed *Reports*, 1921–57.
National Amateur Rowing Association – *Minutes*, 1890–1914; 1945–56.
NARA *Handbooks*, 1921–39.
Printed *Proceedings of the First, Second and Third Conferences of Amateur Rowing Associations*, 1927, 1928 and 1929.
Joint Report of ARA and NARA, 30 March 1949.
Northern Rowing Association – *Minutes*, 1939–57.
The British Rowing Almanack, 1861–1915; 1920–39; 1946 to present.
(The printed reports of the ARA Provincial Committee, AGM's, the three conferences of 1927, 1928 and 1929 as well as the copies of *The British Rowing Almanack* can also be found at Henley Royal Regatta headquarters.)

Club and regatta minutes, letter books and reports

Durham ARC; Empire RC and Tyne United RC; Exeter ARC; Evesham RC; Falcon RC; Furnivall Sculling Club; Hollingworth Lake RC; Leander Club; London RC; Middlesbrough ABC; Nottingham RC; Stratford-upon-Avon RC; Tees ARC; Thames RC; Tyne ARC; Wansbeck, later Cambois RC; Weybridge RC.
Durham Regatta; Henley Royal Regatta; Metropolitan Regatta; Tideway Boxing Day Charity Regatta.
(The *Minutes* of the Falcon, Nottingham and Stratford clubs are held in the local county archives and those of the Boxing Day Charity Regatta at ARA headquarters. All the others can be seen by request from the club or regatta secretaries.)

Official documents

The Public Schools Commission (Clarendon Report), 1864.
The Schools Inquiry Commission (Taunton Report), 1868.
Hansard – Parliamentary Debates, 1937.

Select bibliography

Club histories

C. M. Ainslie, *History of the Falcon Rowing Club* (Typescript, 1969, Oxford City Libraries).

Anonymous, *Rowing at Westminster from 1813 to 1883* (London, 1890).

Anonymous, *Walton R.C.* (privately printed, 1977).

Anonymous, *The Record of the Rowing Club of St Philip and St James, Oxford, 1889–1909* (Oxford, 1910).

C. S. Bell, *Derby Rowing Club – The First Hundred Years, 1879–1979* (Derby, 1979).

H. Bond, *A History of Trinity Hall Boat Club* (Cambridge, 1930).

R. D. Burnell and H. R. N. Rickett, *A Short History of Leander Club, 1818–1963* (Henley-on-Thames, 1968).

A. Davis, *Records of the Marlow Rowing Club, 1871–1921* (Marlow, 1921).

J. Gretton, *et al. Derwent Rowing Club – Centenary 1857–1957* (Derby, 1957).

W. A. Locan, *The Agecroft Story* (Salford, 1960).

London RC, *From Strength to Strength – 1856–1981: Portrait of London R.C.* (London, 1981).

J. A. King, *A Short History of Kingston Rowing Club, 1858–1983* (London, 1981).

W. W. Rouse Ball, *A History of First Trinity Boat Club* (Cambridge 1908).

H. R. Smith, *Dark Blue and White – The History of Evesham Rowing Club* (Evesham, 1948).

K. Tarbuck, ed., *Liverpool Victoria, 1884–1934 – Jubilee Souvenir* (privately printed, 1934).

Typescripts, manuscripts and miscellaneous

W. H. Allnult, *Notes on the Oxford Royal Regatta, 1841–1891* (undated, Oxford City Libraries).

Dora Falconer, *Women's University Rowing between World Wars I and II* (undated, ARA headquarters, London).

John Johnson Collection, 'Regattas and rowing', *Bodleian Library, Box Sport 13.*

R. W. Lee, *Oxford University and Colleges Servants Rowing Club: Centenary Handbook, 1850–1950* (undated, Oxford City Libraries).

John Lehmann, *R. C. Lehmann in America* (in possession of author).

N. Wigglesworth, *A Short History of Rowing in Lancaster* (undated, ARA headquarters).

Newspapers and periodicals

Badminton Magazine of Sports and Pastimes; Bell's Sporting Life in London; The Cambridge Magazine; Cambridge Review; Durham County Advertiser; Exeter Express and Echo; The Field; Fortnightly Review; Fraser's Magazine; Gentlemen's Magazine; Granta; Illustrated London News; Newcastle Daily Chronicle; Newcastle Evening Chronicle; Newcastle Courant; Newcastle Journal; New Liberal Review; Nineteenth Century And After; The Oarsman; Oxford Chronicle; Punch; Rowing Magazine; The Spectator; the Sportsman; Stratford-upon-Avon Herald; The Times; Truth; York Herald.

Books

Rowing

An Amateur, *The Aquatic Oracle or Record of Rowing from 1825 to 1851* (London, 1851).

Anonymous – A member of CUBC, *Aquatic Notes* (Cambridge, 1852).

Anonymous (A. T. W. Shadwell), *The Oarsman, Principles of Rowing* (London, 1846).

Argonaut, E. D. Brickwood, *The Arts of Rowing and Training* (London, 1866).

G. C. Bourne, *A Text-Book of Oarsmanship* (London, 1925).

G. C. Bourne, *Memories of an Eton Wet-Bob of the Seventies* (London, 1933).

E. D. Brickwood, *Boat-Racing: Or the Arts of Rowing and Training* (London, 1876).

F. Brittain, *Oar, Scull and Rudder: A Bibliography of Rowing* (London, 1930).

R. D. Burnell, *Swing Together: Thoughts on Rowing* (London, 1952).

R. D. Burnell, *Henley Regatta – A History* (London, 1957).

R. D. Burnell, *Henley Royal Regatta – A Celebration* (London, 1989).

R. D. Burnell, *The Oxford and Cambridge Boat Race* (London, 1954).

L. S. R. Byrne and E. L. Churchill, *The Eton Book of the River* (Eton, 1935).

L. Cecil-Smith, *Annals of Public School Rowing* (Oxford, 1920).

H. Cleaver, *A History of Rowing* (London, 1957).

T. A. Cook, *Rowing at Henley* (London, 1919).

A. Crump, *A History of Amateur Rowing on the River Lee* (London, 1913).

R. J. Davis, *Boating at Worcester in the Nineteenth Century* (Worcester, undated).

C. Dodd, *Henley Royal Regatta* (London, 1981).

G. C. Drinkwater and T. R. B. Saunders, *The University Boat Race – Official Centenary History, 1829–1929* (London, 1929).

Ian Fairbairn, *Steve Fairbairn on Rowing* (London, 1951).

Steve Fairbairn, *Chats on Rowing* (London, 1934).

P. Haig-Thomas and M. A. Nicholson, *The English Style of Rowing* (London, 1958).

Iota, *The Boat-Racing Calendar or Record of the Performances of the Principal Winning Amateurs in England and Wales from 1835 to 1857* (London, 1858).

R. C. Lehmann, *Rowing* (London, 1898).

R. C. Lehmann, *The Complete Oarsman* (London, 1908).

A. A Macfarlane-Grieve, *A History of Durham Rowing* (Newcastle upon Tyne, 1922).

A. Maclaren, *Training in Theory and Practice* (London, first ed. 1866, second ed. 1874).

W. J. Macmichael, *The Oxford and Cambridge Boat Races* (Cambridge, 1870).

R. Meldrum, *Rowing and Coaching: Notes on One of the Fine Arts* (London, 1950).

R. Meldrum, *Rowing to a Finish* (London, 1955).

J. E. Morgan, *University Oars, Being a Critical Enquiry into the After Health of the Men who Rowed in the Oxford and Cambridge Boat Race, 1829–1869* (London, 1873).

K. Osborne, *Boat Racing in Britain, 1715–1975* (London, 1975).

R. P. P. Rowe and C. M. Pitman, *Rowing* (London, 1898).

W. E. Sherwood, *Oxford Rowing* (Oxford and London 1900).

The Sportsman, British Sports and Sportsmen – Yachting and Rowing (London, 1916).

H. T. Steward, *Henley Royal Regatta, 1939–1902* (London, 1903).

G. G. T. Treherne and J. H. D. Goldie, *Record of the University Boat Race, 1929–1883*

(London, 1884).

E. Warre, 'Athletics or physical exercise and recreation', Pt. I, X, General Hygiene, The Health Exhibition Literature (London, 1884).

E. Warre, On the Grammar of Rowing (Oxford, 1909).

W. B. Woodgate, Boating (London, 1888).

General

Anonymous, Frederick James Furnivall – A Volume of Personal Records (London, 1911).

N. Annan, Leslie Stephen (London, 1951).

P. Bailey, Leisure and Class in Victorian England: Rational Recreations and the Contest for Control, 1830–1885 (London, 1978).

M. Baker, The Rise of the Victorian Actor (London, 1978).

G. Best, Mid-Victorian Britain, 1851–75 (London, 1971).

D. Birley, The Willow Wand – Some Cricket Myths Explored (London, 1979).

R. Brimley-Johnson, The Undergraduate – From Dr. Christopher Wordsworth's 'A Social Life at the English Universities' in the Eighteenth Century (London, 1928).

W. L. Burn, The Age of Equipoise (London, 1964).

R. A. Church, Economic and Social Change in a Midland Town: Victorian Nottingham, 1815–1900 (London, 1966).

T. A. Cook, The Sunlit Hours – A Record of Sport and Life (London, 1925).

T. A. Cook and G. Nickalls, Thomas Doggett Deceased – A Famous Comedian (London, 1908).

C. Crawley, Trinity Hall – The History of a Cambridge College, 1350–1975 (Cambridge, 1977).

C. Dickens, junior, Dictionary of the Thames (London, 1972 ed.).

E. Dunning and K. Sheard, Barbarians, Gentlemen and Players – A Sociological Study of the Development of Rugby Football (Oxford, 1979).

G. Faber, Jowett – Portrait with Background (London, 1957).

V. H. H. Green, Oxford Common Room – A Study of Lincoln College and Mark Pattison (London, 1957).

V. H. H. Green, The Commonwealth of Lincoln College, 1427–1977 (Oxford, 1977).

K. Gregson, Corvan – A Victorian Entertainer and His Songs (Banbury, 1983).

D. Haig-Thomas, I Leaped before I Looked – Sport at Home and Abroad (London, 1936).

H. Harris, Under Oars – Reminiscences of a Thames Lighterman (London, 1978).

G. Hill, History of the Tyne Lodge, 1863–1913 (Newcastle-on-Tyne, 1913).

R. Holt, Sport and the British – A Modern History (Oxford, 1989).

J. R. de S. Honey, Tom Brown's Universe – The Development of the Victorian Public School (London, 1977).

M. R. James, Eton and King's: Recollections, Mostly Trivial (London, 1926).

A. Kingsley, Ravenshoe (London, 1894 ed.).

R. Latham and W. Matthews, eds., The Diary of Samuel Pepys (London, 1970 ed.).

O. MacDonagh, Early Victorian Government (London, 1977).

E. Mack and W. H. G. Armytage, Thomas Hughes (London, 1952).

F. W. Maitland, The Life and Letters of Leslie Stephen (London, 1906).

J. A. Mangan, Athleticism in the Victorian and Edwardian Public Schools (Cambridge, 1981).

R. B. Mansfield, *The Log of the Water Lily During Three Cruises* (London, 1873).
R. B. Martin, *The Dust of Combat: A Life of Charles Kingsley* (London, 1959).
Tony Mason, *Association Football and English Society, 1863–1915* (Sussex, 1980).
Tony Mason, *Sport in Britain* (London, 1988).
D. Newsome, *Godliness and Good Learning* (London, 1961).
D. Newsome, ed., *Edwardian Excursions – From the Diaries of A. C. Benson, 1898–1904* (London, 1981).
J. H. Newman, *The Idea of a University* (Oxford, 1976 ed.).
G. Nickalls, *Life's a Pudding, An Autobiography* (London, 1939).
G. O. Nickalls, *A Rainbow in the Sky – Reminiscences* (London, 1974).
M. Prior, *Fisher Row – Fishermen, Bargemen and Canal Boatmen in Oxford, 1500–1900* (Oxford, 1982).
S. Rothblatt, *The Revolution of the Dons – Cambridge and Society in Victorian England* (London, 1968).
M. Sherman, *Athletics and Football* (London, third ed., 1889).
Stonehenge, *British Rural Sports* (London, 1861).
J. Strutt, *The Sports and Pastimes of the People of England* (London, 1801).
F. M. L. Thompson, *The Rise of Respectable Society – A Social History of Victorian Britain, 1830–1900* (London, 1988).
G. M. Trevelyan, *An Autobiography and other Essays* (London, 1949).
A. Trollope, ed., *British Sports and Pastimes* (London, 1868).
W. Tuckwell, *Reminiscences of Oxford* (London, 1900).
J. Walvin, *The People's Game* (London, 1975).
M. J. Wiener, *English Culture and the Decline of the Industrial Spirits, 1850–1980* (Cambridge, 1982).
J. Wilson, *Tyneside Songs and Drolleries* (Newcastle upon Tyne, 1890).
W. B. Woodgate, *Reminiscences of an Old Sportsman* (London, 1909).

Articles

J. W. Fewster, 'The Keelmen of Tyneside in the eighteenth century', *Durham University Journal*, New Series, XIX, 1957–8.
J. W. Fewster, 'The last struggles of the Tyneside keelmen', *Durham University Journal*, New Series, XXIV, 1962–3.
K. Gregson, 'When the boat comes in – the songs of nineteenth sport', *English Dance and Song*, Winter 1978.
K. Gregson, 'Songs of Tyneside boat racing', *Bulletin of the North East Groups for the study of Labour History*, 16, 1982.
K. Gregson, 'Champions at Talkin Tarn', *Cumbria Magazine*, 32, no. 6, 1982.
E. Halladay, 'Of pride and prejudice: the amateur question in nineteenth century English rowing', *International Journal of the History of Sport*, 4, no. 1, May 1987.
W. F. Mandle, 'The professional cricketer in England in the nineteenth century', *Labour History*, XXIII, 1972.
T. C. Mendenhall, 'Coaches and coaching (V) – the British are coming (R. C. Lehmann)', *The Oarsman*, January/February 1979.
A. Metcalfe, 'Organised sport in the mining communities of south Nothumberland, 1800–1889', *Victorian Studies*, 25, no. 4, Summer 1982.
N. Wigglesworth, 'A History of rowing in the North West of England', *British*

Journal of Sports History, 3, 1986.

Unpublished theses

H. R. Harrington, *Muscular Christianity – A Study of a Victorian Idea* (Ph.D. thesis, Stanford University, USA, 1971).

N. Wigglesworth, *Rowing in the North West* (M.Ed. thesis, Manchester University, 1983).

Index

Addy, M., 12, 15
Agecroft RC, 60, 69, 70, 151, 157, 158, 161, 177, 178
Amateur Athletics Association, 3, 86
Amateur Athletics Club, 3
Amateur Rowing Association, 3–5, 90, 91–2, 108, 109, 117, 120, 121–2, 139, 141–2, 145, 148, 149, 160, 161, 167, 168, 169, 179, 190
  amateur definition, 84–5, 94, 120, 126, 172, 187
  coxed four issue, 179
  foundation, 83
  Henley, 84–5, 87, 114–16
  National Amateur Rowing Association, 89, 92–3, 97, 145, 170–4, 183–9
  nominating clubs, 180, 186–9, 191
  Olympic Regattas, 117–22, 124, 141–2, 183
  women's rowing, 153, 187–8, 190
amateurism
  ARA definition, 84–5, 94, 120, 126, 172, 187
  Brickwood's definition, 75–6
  Egan on, 74–5
  foreign competition, 5, 108–22 passim, 171, 183–4, 186–7
  Henley definition, 81–2
  NARA definition, 88–9, 142, 145–6
  Putney definition, 79–80, 81

universities, 43–6
Almanack, British Rowing, 83, 86, 174, 181, 185
Ampthill, Lord, 133, 134
Ancholme RC, 183
Aquatic Oracle, 31–8
Argonauts, 57
Ariel RC, 61, 77
Arnold, F. M., 203
Association Football, 2, 25–6
Atalanta Club, USA, 108, 206
athleticism, 44, 48, 50–1, 53
athletics, 3–4, 9, 46–7, 86–7
Aylings, oarmakers, 208

Babcock, J. C., 205
Bailey, P., 1–2, 4
Balfour, E. R., 216
Balliol College, Oxford, 49, 54
Barn Cottage, 190
Barnes, 28, 144
Barry, E., 26, 144, 175
Barry, H. A., 26, 28, 185
Barry RC, 91
Beach, W., 24
Bell's Life, 11, 29, 74–5, 77, 80, 200
Beresford, J. (Senior), 134, 135
Beresford, J. (Junior), 126, 184
Besant, W., 2
Bideford, 150
Biffen, W., 23
Birch, R. O., 205
Birmingham, RC, 149
Blackstaffe, H. T., 169

boatbuilders
  Clasper, H., 198–200
  Clasper, J. H., 15, 209
  Jewett, R., 57, 200, 206
  Noulton and Maynard, 14
  Pocock, W., 4
  Taylor, M., 15, 58, 200, 201
  Wentzell and Cownden, 199
  Winship, T., 15
boating, 71–2
boat design, 197–209 *passim*
Boat Race, 31–2, 33, 44, 54, 55, 124, 127–8, 135, 136, 137–8, 193, 197, 200, 206, 212–15
Boat Racing Calendar, 31–8
Bolton and Ringley RC, 74, 75, 76
Bourne, G. C., 127, 128–30, 136, 201–2, 203–4, 206–7, 208
Bourne RC, 170
Bowen R., 53
Bradley, M., 130
Brasenose College, Oxford, 47, 52
Brickwood, E. D., 29, 30, 55, 56, 75–6, 79, 80, 202–3
Briggs, J., 176
Bristowe, Rev. C. J., 87
British ARA, 185, 188
British Olympic Association, 118, 183
British Rowing Board, 174, 184
Brown, A., 198
Brown, W., 205
Bruce, S. M., 129, 132
Buccleugh, Duke of, 11
Bucknall, H. C., 28
Burnell, R. D., 130, 185, 206
Burton-on-Trent, 91, 149

Cambridge University BC, 32, 50, 115–16, 124, 125, 127–8, 130, 184, 185, 192, 200, 201, 202, 203, 204, 206, 207
  Boat Race (1858), 213–14, 216
  early rowing, 44
  Fairbairn style, 131, 136
  inter-war years, 126–7, 135–6
  Putney rules, 79
  watermen coaches, 46

Cambridge Subscription Rooms, 47, 57
Cambridgeshire ARA, 145
Cambois RC, *see* Wansbeck RC
Campbell, C., 11, 30
Canadian Association of American Oarsmen, 119
Candlish, J., 13
Carlisle, Earl of, 11
Casamajor, A. A., 9, 57, 77, 204
Cecil Ladies BC, 153
Central Council for Physical Recreation, 179
Cercle Nautique de France, 80, 109
Chambers, R., 11, 15, 19–21, 23, 182, 204, 205, 219, 220–3
Cheltenham College, 52
Chester-le-Street RC, 27, 179, 182
Chinnery, Walter and Harry, 25
Christ Church, Oxford, 44, 52, 127–8
Civil Service Ladies RC, 154
Clarendon Report (1864), 29
Clasper, H., 11, 13, 14–15, 17, 18–21, 22, 23, 28, 30, 42, 60, 182, 201, 219, 223
  Five Brothers, 198–9
  oars, 207–8
  outriggers, 198
  style, 204, 207
  training, 216–17
Clasper, J. H., 15, 204–5, 206, 209
Clasper, Richard, 13
Clasper, Robert, 12
Close, John and James, 70, 74
Club Nautique de Gand, Belgium, 111–12, 117, 125
club subscriptions, 154–5
Clydesdale RC, 68
coastal rowing, 143, 145
Columbia College, USA, 80, 82
Conan Doyle, Sir Arthur, 118
Conant, J. W., 200
Coombes, R., 18–19, 198–9, 207, 217
Cook, T. A., 115, 118
Cornell University, USA, 84, 111, 115
Corsair Club, 61

Corvan, E., 220–3
Cotton, G. E. L., 29, 51
Cotton, H. B., 216
Courtney, G., 111
Cowen, J., 12
Cox, G. V., 8
cricket, 2, 131–2

Dart ARC, 150
Dartmouth ARC, 150
de Coubertin, Baron Pierre, 109, 110
de Havilland, R. S., 54, 55, 128
Denman, G., 12
Derby Grammar School, 52, 153
Derby RC, 69, 152, 157, 160, 161, 168
Derwent RC, 153–4
Desborough, Lord, see Grenfell, W. H.
Desborough Cup, 159, 169
Deva Club, 91
Dickens, C. (Junior), 71
diet, 212–13, 215, 217
Doggett's Coat and Badge, 8, 26, 187, 198
Dolphin Club, 43, 45, 80
Dublin University, 83
Dudley Ward, W., 115
Durham
  Dean and Chapter, 70
  school, 38, 52
  university 70
  see also regattas
Durham ARC, 58, 69, 94
  Durham Regatta, 60
  local goodwill, 70
  membership, 72–3, 96–7, 153
  subscriptions, 155
Durham University BC, 38, 93, 198

Eagers, E., 12
Edwards-Moss, Sir John, 54, 112, 114
Edwards-Moss, T. C., 207
Egan, T. S., 24, 47, 48, 50, 54, 55, 57, 62, 68, 77, 79, 120, 131, 139, 146, 180, 186, 192, 193, 203, 204, 213–14, 216
  amateur issue, 74–5, 76

creed, 46
Emmett, F., 198
Empire (and Commonwealth) Games, 120–1, 187, 188
Empire RC, 27, 176, 177, 178, 182
Escombe, F. J., 130, 136
Eton College, 8, 28, 30, 51–2, 53, 111, 130, 137, 197, 202, 203, 206–7, 208, 209
Eton Vilkings, 126
European Rowing Championships, 117, 184, 188
Evesham RC, 60, 94, 160, 175, 177, 178
  local goodwill, 70–1
  membership, 72, 151, 153
  subscriptions, 155
Exeter ARC, 72, 147, 150–1, 153, 178
  local goodwill, 72
  membership, 152
  women's rowing, 154
Exeter College, Oxford, 46–7, 51, 198, 200, 202
Eyre, W. H., 59, 133, 134, 169, 171, 206

Fairbairn, S., 125, 128, 129, 131, 135–6, 137, 138, 139, 142, 145, 158, 159–60, 169
Fairbairn style, 129–30, 131–2, 135–6, 138, 190
Fairrie, J., 201
Falcon RC, 143, 152, 161
Farnell, L. R., 51
Fawcus, W., 37
Fédération Internationale des Sociétés d'Aviron, 117, 119–20, 183–4, 188
Field, The, 85, 86–7, 90–1, 92, 111, 113, 118
Fisher Row, Oxford, 7
fixed rowlocks, 130
Fletcher, W. A. L., 127
fouling, 21–5, 31, 32, 45, 59
Frankfurt RC, Germany, 108
Freeman, H. A., 205
Fry, C. B., 131–2
Furnivall, Dr F. J., 87–9, 90, 200

Furnivall Sculling Club, 88, 153, 154, 162, 179, 189
  subscriptions, 155
  war damage, 177, 178
Funny Club, 31

Gateshead and District RC, 27, 178
Gibbon, J. H., 136
Gold, Sir Harcourt, 121, 183
Goldie, J. H. D., 205
Gonville and Caius, Cambridge, 208
Grace, Dr W. G., 2
Green, R. A. W., 209
Greenall, R., 203
Grenfell, W. H., 112–16, 121, 125, 170, 173
Grosvenor RC, 59
Gulston, R. S., 206

Haig-Thomas, David, 125–6
Haig-Thomas, Peter, 130, 136
Hampshire and Dorset ARA, 143, 145
Hanlan, E., 24, 207
Harvard University, USA, 114, 117
Hastie, J., 134
Hawthorn RC, 27, 178
Head of the River Race, 157, 159–60, 181
Henley Royal Regatta, 3, 4, 31, 33, 37, 52, 54, 55, 56, 58, 61, 74–5, 87, 93, 94, 97, 121, 124, 126, 131, 135, 137, 149, 156, 170, 180, 183, 186–7, 189, 193, 200, 205, 206
  amateur issue, 80–2
  ARA, 84–5, 87
  coxed fours, 179–80
  foreign entries, 5, 67, 80–2, 108–16, 117, 120, 171, 183
  Peace Regatta (1919), 120, 145, 167
  regatta (1878), 80, 108
  seven-oar race (1843), 47, 48
  stewards, 4, 67, 76, 80–2, 85, 109–16, 121, 173
  universities, 61–2, 126–7
Henley RC, 58, 91
Hereford RC, 160

Hewett, W. A. S., 90, 92
Hillside Club, USA, 83–4
Hogg, Quintin, 87
Hollingworth Lake, 71–2
Hop Bitter Company, 12
Hornby, J. J., 53
horse-racing, 9
Hughes, G., 48
Hughes, T., 47, 48, 88
Hutt, W., 12

Ilex RC, 61
inns and hostelries, 12–13
internal combustion engine, 158
international rowing, 5, 80–2, 108–22 passim, 124–5, 156, 171, 178, 183–4, 186–7, 190–1
Ipswich, 145
Irex Club, 91
Iveagh, Lord, 28, 170

Jackson, H., 50
James, M. R., 50
Janousek, B., 190
Jarrow, 144, 150
Jerome, J. K., 71
Jesus College, Cambridge, 52, 128, 130, 131, 137, 215
Jewitt, R., 57, 200, 206
Johnson, S. H., 186
John O'Gaunt RC, 58–9, 94, 205
joint co-ordinating committee (ARA/NARA), 173–4, 184–6
Jowett, B., 49

Kean, E., 10
Keate, Dr J., 51
Keble College, Oxford, 69
Kelley, H., 11, 13, 19, 20, 21–2, 23–4, 207, 223
keelmen, 7, 14–15, 24–5
keelless boats, 199–202, 204
Kennedy, B. H., 52
Kidd, Rev. B. J., 68–9
Kilmorey, Earl of, 11
King's College, Cambridge, 50
Kingsley, H., 28
Kingsley, C., 47–8, 50, 88

Kingston RC (Hull), 148
Kingston RC, 61, 79, 115, 125, 126, 149, 189

Lady Margaret BC, Cambridge, 45, 73, 130
Lancaster RC, 58–9, 60
Lea ARA, 90, 145
Leander Club, 57, 112, 114, 115–16, 125, 135, 176, 185, 187, 190, 191, 203
  boathouse, 149
  fouling, 31, 32
  foundation and early days, 8, 30, 56
  professionals, 10–11
  Putney rules, 79
  university connection, 59, 115, 126
  wagers, 43, 44–5
le Blanc Smith, S., 91
Lee, G. W., 80, 111
Lehmann, R. C., 81, 120, 125, 127, 139, 142, 145, 203, 208, 216
  foreign competition, 113–14, 118, 119
  Harvard, 114
  professional definition, 91–3
Leicester RC, 91, 94
Liddell, H. G., 52
Lincoln College, Oxford, 49
Linden RC, 177
Littledale, J. B., 201–2
Liverpool Victoria RC, 149–50, 152, 153
London RC, 12, 24, 25, 61, 62, 67, 68, 72, 112, 115, 125, 126, 128, 133, 135, 149, 159, 176, 187, 205
  boathouse, 149
  foundation, 57–8, 76
  international competition, 78–9, 108, 109, 115, 157
  Metropolitan regatta, 77–8
  Metropolitan Rowing Association and Amateur Rowing Association, 83–5
  perceived role, 77–8

Putney rules, 79–80, 108
longitudinal oscillation, 201
Lowndes, J., 73
Lyon's Subscription Room, 11, 30
Lythgoe, I., 69
Lyttelton, E., 132

Maclaren, A., 213–5
McLean, D. H., 208
Maddison, H., 23
Magdalen College, School, 52
Magdalen College, Oxford, 134
Manchester Grammar School, 153
manual labour clause, 3, 80, 81, 84, 91, 170–2
Marlow RC, 91
Marylebone Cricket Club, 75
masonic order, 11
Maynard, G., 14
Maurice, Dr F. D., 47–8, 50, 88
Meldrum, R., 130
Menzies, F., 203
Merifield, G. J. P., 157, 176
Merivale, C., 44
Mersey RC, 94
Merton College, Oxford, 169
Messenger, J., 22
Metropolitan Police RC, 173
Metropolitan Rowing Association, 83
Midland ARA, 149
Middlesbrough ABC, 75, 144, 150, 151, 155, 175, 178
Mid-Tyne RC, 150
Molesey BC, 125, 189
Morgan, E. H., 52
Morgan, H. A., 52, 215
Morgan, J. E., 51, 214–15
muscular Christianity, 16, 48, 160
music halls, 219–23 *passim*

National Amateur Rowing Association, 3–5, 89–91, 93, 108, 113, 121, 141, 142, 144, 148, 150, 152, 159, 161, 169, 174
  amateur definition, 88–9, 142, 145–6

Amateur Rowing Association, 89, 92–3, 97, 120, 145, 170–4, 183–9
  conferences (1927, 1928, 1929), 145–7, 155, 167
  demise, 188–9
  membership, 142–4
  Olympic regattas, 118, 119–20
  Peace Regatta (1919), 120, 145, 167
  professional issue, 86, 142–3, 175–7, 181–3
National Fitness Campaign, 148, 174–7, 183
National Provincial Bank RC, 177
National Water Sports Centre, 190
Nemesis RC, 153
Nereus, Holland, 110
Newark RC, 178
Newcastle Christmas Handicap, 28, 144, 159, 175
Newcastle Chronicle, 12
Newcastle RC, 37, 62, 150
Newcastle Royal Grammar School, 153
New College, Oxford, 52, 70, 112, 137
Newell, R., 18, 21, 199
New Zealand ARA, 146
Newman, Cardinal J. H., 48
Nicholson, M. A., 130
Nickalls, G. O., 121, 162, 180–1, 183–4, 187–9
Nickalls, Guy, 54, 118, 121, 124, 127
Nisbet, R. A., 135
nominating clubs, 180, 186–9, 191
North East/Northern Rowing Council, 93, 108, 169
Northern Athletics Association, 3
Northern RC, 30, 150
Northern Rowing Association, 176, 181–2, 186, 189
Norwich ARA, 145
Nottidge, J., 57, 76–7, 83
Nottingham BC, 160
Nottingham RC, 29–30, 68, 155, 159, 160
Nottingham and Union RC, 121, 156
Noulton, W., 14, 31, 45

oars, 207–8
Oatlands RC, 151
Olympic Regattas, 117–22, 124, 145, 156, 167, 170–1, 178, 183–4, 186, 191
Ooms, J. K., 110
orthodox style, 54, 55, 127–30, 133, 138, 142, 190, 204
outriggers, 47, 198–9, 202, 208
Oxford ARA, 143, 145
Oxford Subscription Rooms, 57
Oxford University BC, 24, 54, 55, 124, 125, 127, 130, 185, 192, 198, 200–1, 202, 203
  Boat Race (1858), 213–14
  foreign competition, 116
  inter-war years, 136
  Putney rules, 79
  watermen coaches, 46, 204, 212
Oxford University and Colleges Servants RC, 68
Oxford Vacation Club, 73
Oxo Cup, 28

Page, J. H., 180–1, 184, 187–9, 191
Palmerston RC, 61, 77
Paris Exhibition Regatta (1867), 79, 80, 108
Parish, J., 31, 45
Patterson, W., 13
Pattison, M., 49
Payne, K. M., 136
pedestrianism, 9, 16–17
Pembroke College, Cambridge, 137, 206
Pengwern RC, 117
Pennsylvania University, USA, 112, 114–15
Pepys, S., 7
Phelps, E., 26
Philadelphia Centennial Regatta (1876), 79, 80, 108, 111
Physical Training and Recreation Act (1937), 174
Pitman, C. M., 172, 207, 215
Playford, F., 57, 108, 207
Playford, H. H., 24, 25, 57, 81
Pocock, W., 199

Port Royal ARC, 150–1, 178
Probert, Prebendary P. S. G., 87,
   145, 167
professional rowing
   apprentice races, 10, 11, 22
   decline, 10–11, 24–8
   fouling, 21–4
   gambling, 21, 22–3
   inns and hostelries, 12–14, 15, 26
   north-eastern clubs, 27–8, 144,
      150, 175–6, 181–3
   patronage, 9–12, 25, 26
   Thames clubs, 28, 144, 175, 181–3
Provincial Amateur Rowing
      Council, 93, 121, 148, 155,
      157, 160, 161, 179–80, 185–6,
      188
pugilism, 9
Putney rules, 79–80, 81, 83, 108, 153

Radley College, 52, 53, 137
railways, 17–18, 68, 157–8
rational recreation, 16
Reading RC, 149
regattas
   Agecroft, 60, 72, 74, 75, 76
   Barnes and Mortlake, 96
   Bedford, 86, 189
   Burton, 169
   Chester, 32, 37, 42
   Derby, 60, 157
   Durham, 27, 28, 32, 37, 42, 56, 60,
      70, 73, 144, 148, 181–3
   Evesham, 60, 71, 85, 86, 154, 157,
      169
   Greenwich, 8
   Interim, 159
   King's Lynn, 205
   Lancaster, 74, 157
   Maidenhead, 94
   Manchester and Salford, 60
   Marlow, 189
   Metropolitan, 61, 77–8, 83
   Nottingham, 157
   Oxford Royal, 73, 143, 169
   Reading, 59, 168, 189
   Roundhay Park, 75
   St Neots, 189

Sons of the Thames, 25
Southampton, 86
Stratford-upon-Avon, 85, 86, 169
Talkin Tarn, 11, 37
Tideway Boxing Day Charity,
      144, 159, 162, 169–70, 175
Thames, Royal Thames and
      Thames National, 18–19, 33,
      76–7, 199
Tewkesbury, 85
Tyne, 59, 179, 199
Wallingford, 189
Wargrave, 85, 154
Worcester, 37, 60, 61, 85, 86, 157
Windermere, 4
York, 60–1, 157, 182
   see also Henley Royal Regatta
Regent Street Polytechnic, 87
Renforth, J., 15, 19–21, 79, 182, 205,
      206, 219, 223
Renforth, S., 15
Rew, C., 139
Ridley, G., 19, 220, 223
Risley, R. W., 202
river by-laws, 47
Rogers, G., 185
Ross RC, 153
Royal and Ancient Golf Club, 74
Royal Chester RC, 58, 62, 86, 115,
      125, 149, 178, 200, 201, 207
Rowe, R. P. P., 207, 215
Rowing Magazine, 187, 190
Rudge family, 70
Rugby League, 3
Rugby Union, 2–3, 50
Runcorn RC, 72
Ryton RC, 62, 150

sabbath rowing, 69–71, 160–1
Sadler, J., 23–4, 206
Sadler, W., 205
St James' Gazette, 216
St John's College, Oxford, 111, 200
St Philip and St. James's RC, 68–9,
      162
St Thomas RC, 150
Scottish Rowing Association, 174,
      184, 185

Selwyn, C. J., 45, 50, 62, 79, 120, 131, 139, 146, 180, 186, 192, 193
Shadwell, A. T. W., 47, 50, 62, 68, 79, 120, 131, 139, 146, 180, 186, 192, 193
  Boat Race, 203, 212–13, 213–14, 216
  creed and influence, 46, 55
  cox of seven-oar, 48
  Eton coach, 53
  orthodox style, 54, 204
Shafto, C. D., 97
Shaw, A. B., 90, 92
Shoe-wae-cae-mette crew, USA, 80
Shrewsbury School, 52, 137
Skey, F. C., 214
Skiff Racing Association, 97
sliding seat, 24, 54, 133, 204–7
South Hylton RC, 27
South Shields RC, 150
Southampton University College, 171
Sportsman, 12, 26, 78
Stephen, L., 47–50, 55
Stourport RC, 178
Stratford-upon-Avon RC, 151–2, 155, 158, 161, 178
Stretch, T. H. E., 216
Strutt, J., 7–8
Stuart, D. C. R., 127–8, 129
styles in rowing, 127–39 *passim*, 203–9
Swann, Rev. S., 87, 171
swivel rowlocks, 130, 133, 208–9
Sydney RC, Australia, 117

Talkin Tarn, 11, 200
Taunton Report (1968), 39
Taylor, J., 205, 206, 209
Taylor, M., 9, 15, 200, 201, 202, 204, 205, 207, 212, 214
Tees ABC, 94, 144, 154, 159, 161, 175, 178
  membership, 151, 152, 153
  pleasure boating, 72
Tees ARC, 178, 179
television, 193

Ten Eyck, E. H., 110
Thames ARA, 144, 145, 159
Thames RC, 61, 84, 87, 110, 111, 112, 115, 125, 126, 128, 133, 134–5, 139, 159, 184, 205
  boathouse, 149
  membership, 59
  Putney rules, 79
Thames Rowing Council, 93
Thames Subscription Room, 76–7
Thames Tradesmen's RC, 181, 190, 191
Thring, E., 29, 51
Tideway Scullers School, 190
Times, The, 10, 23, 79, 83, 120, 129, 138, 171, 173
Tradesmen's Rowing Club Association, 144, 154, 159, 169, 175, 182
Trent RC, 91
Trevelyan, G. M., 88
Trickett, E., 11, 12, 24
Trinity College, Cambridge, 45, 50
Trinity Hall, Cambridge, 48–9, 88, 111, 126, 200
Truth, 91, 92
Tuckwell, W., 47
Tugwell, C., 144, 145–7, 169
  Amateur Rowing Association negotiations, 171–2, 183–9
  National Fitness Council, 174–7
  professional clubs, 175–6, 181–3
Tyne ARC, 30, 31, 58, 62, 70, 96–7, 144, 155, 160, 177–9
  membership, 150, 153
Tyne United RC, 37, 150
Tynemouth RC, 37, 150
Twickenham RC, 115, 189

unaffiliated clubs, 93–4, 144, 148
Union des Sociétés Françaises des Sports Athlétiques, 109
University College, Oxford, 53
University of London, 154, 190, 192
universities (Oxford and Cambridge)
  early rowing, 8–9, 28, 44–5, 47
  East-end missions, 88, 90

educational aims, 48–9
games, 50–1, 136
Henley, 61–2, 126–7
public schools, 44, 53, 55
watermen, 44, 45–6
see also Boat Race

Vaughan, C., 51
Vesper BC, USA, 116
Vesta RC, 169
Vincent, F. J., 73, 89

Wachusetts BC, USA, 110
Waddington, W. H., 109
Walker RC, 27, 178
Wallace, J., 200
Wallasey Grammar School, 153
Wallsend RC, 27, 178
Walton RC, 151
Wandle Club, 57
Wansbeck RC, 27–8, 152, 160, 176
Warner, P. F., 132
Warre, Dr E., 53–5, 125, 128, 132,
    201, 202, 203–4, 208, 209, 212,
    216
  foreign competition, 81–2,
    112–16, 121
  orthodox style, 54, 55, 129

Warwick BC, 92, 155
West of England ARA, 143, 145, 146,
    150, 157, 168
Westminster School, 28, 51–2, 197
Wetherel, W. P., 91
Weybridge RC, 144, 145, 150, 151,
    154, 156, 159, 169, 174–5, 177
Wharton family, 70
White, T., 220–3
Williams, D., 183, 185
Wilson, J., 16, 19, 220–1, 223
Wingfield Sculls, 28, 31, 32, 37, 43,
    73, 75, 170
Winship, T., 205
Wolsencroft, S., 199, 200
women's rowing, 153–4, 169, 187–8,
    190
Woodgate, W. B., 24, 25, 31, 56, 61,
    76, 113, 138, 199, 202, 207,
    209, 215
  amateurism, 42, 47, 75
Worcester RC, 72, 151
Wordsworth, C., 215
World Rowing Championships,
    190–1

Yale University, USA, 111, 115
York City RC, 94, 143